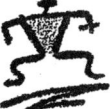

DISCOVER REFLEXOLOGY

ROSALIND OXENFORD

DISCOVER REFLEXOLOGY

ROSALIND OXENFORD

KATHERINE ARMITAGE
Illustrator

Ulysses Press Berkeley, CA
1997

This book has been written and published strictly for informational purposes, and in no way should it be used as a substitute for consultation with your medical doctor or other health care professional. All facts in this book came from medical files, clinical journals, scientific publications, personal interviews, published trade books, self-published materials by experts, magazine articles, and the personal-practice experiences of the authorities quoted or sources cited. You should not consider educational material herein to be the practice of medicine or to replace consultation with a physician or other medical practitioner. The author and publisher are providing you with information in this work so that you can have the knowledge and can choose, at your own risk, to act on that knowledge. The author and publisher also urge all readers to be aware of their health status and to consult health professionals before beginning any health program, including changes in dietary habits.

All names and identifying characteristics of real persons have been changed in the text to protect their confidentiality.

Copyright © 1997 Rosalind Oxenford. All rights reserved under International and Pan-American Copyright Conventions, including the right to reproduce this book or portions thereof in any form whatsoever, except for use by a reviewer in connection with a review.

Published by: Ulysses Press
P.O. Box 3440
Berkeley, CA 94703-3440

Library of Congress Catalog Card Number: 97-60159

ISBN: 1-56975-112-9

Printed in the United States by George Banta Company

10 9 8 7 6 5 4 3 2 1

Editorial and production: Leslie Henriques, Claire Chun, Lily Chou, Nicole O'Hay
Cover Design: B & L Design
Indexer: Sayre Van Young
Typesetter: David Wells

Distributed in the United States by Publishers Group West and in Canada by Raincoast Books.

To David with my love.

This book is one of the fruits of the life we have made together.

TABLE OF CONTENTS

Acknowledgments — x

Chapter One
    Health and the Role Reflexology
    Plays in Maintaining It — 1

Chapter Two
    What Is Reflexology? — 9

Chapter Three
    The History of Reflexology — 16

Chapter Four
    How Reflexology Works — 20

Chapter Five
    What Do We Mean by Health? — 24

Chapter Six
    Trauma and Disease — 31

Chapter Seven
    The Effects of Reflexology — 38

Chapter Eight
    The Holistic Approach — 45

Chapter Nine
    What Are You Aiming for
    and Intending To Do? — 49

Chapter Ten
    What You Need to
    Give a Reflexology Treatment — 53

Chapter Eleven
    Foot Massage — 57

Chapter Twelve
    Reflexology Techniques and
    Learning to Give a Treatment   67

Chapter Thirteen
    Knowledge and Wisdom   82

Chapter Fourteen
    The Routine   88

Chapter Fifteen
    Case Studies   99

Recommended Reading   111

Index   114

ACKNOWLEDGMENTS

My thanks go to: Mo who made the writing of the book possible at all by keeping our home together so superbly; Jayne for keeping me together; Jessica, Richard and Thomas, my children, for their encouragement and enthusiasm; Wendy, Mandy and Peter Chappell for understanding sufficiently for me to have the belief to develop my ideas; Tessa for asking me; all my students and patients, who have been as much a part of my learning process as I have been part of theirs; the warm and wise colleagues I have in the Association of Reflexologists, and especially Hazel Goodwin and Jenny Hok, who have given me much support.

HEALTH AND THE ROLE REFLEXOLOGY PLAYS IN MAINTAINING IT

Reflexology has long been used to promote good health and was practiced in ancient China as part of a health-care system based on meridian theory. It was used in conjunction with acupuncture, the feet being worked first to find out which body parts were out of balance or in trouble; to relax and break down congestions; to stimulate the circulation and energy flow; and to enhance all the body systems through stimulation. Acupuncture needles were then applied to specific points to finely tune the system, to free and improve the flow of energy around the body, and to maximize the effectiveness of the treatment.

Pressure point therapy and foot massage have been used the world over for thousands of years, but although we have evidence of this we know little of the understanding behind the work except from China. Knowledge of the body/mind/spirit of human beings was as comprehensive as wisdom was profound in ancient China. Both have been passed down to us today through the principles and practice of acupuncture.

A Holistic Understanding of How We Work

In stark contrast with many modern systems of medicine, reflexology, a holistic therapy, embraces every facet of our existence and makes sense of the interrelationship between the differing areas of our lives, as well as the various systems of our bodies as they work together for our well-being.

If an incident at work has made you so angry that you are seething, your adrenaline is pumping, and your body systems are speeded up, ready for action, this means that your muscles have tensed, your metabolism is working faster to process energy for immediate use, blood is pounding through your body, and your breathing has speeded up. Whether you are able to use up this increased energy and are able to release it by dealing with the situation, or whether you are unable to take action because it may not be appropriate, which causes you to hold on to (store) the added energy, your body reserves will have been depleted by the rush of the high energy–making process.

The body will have certain requirements in order to make good again, or heal itself. The muscles will need to relax, either naturally or with help; your energy reserves will have to be replenished by giving the body more fuel in the form of food; the type of fuel/food will in turn affect the way in which the systems are able to return to normal functioning in the future. If all this happens naturally you will have no problems. If, on the other hand, you continue to feel bottled up all day, snatch a prepackaged sandwich for lunch, rush home via the supermarket to pick up a microwave meal for the evening, and arrive home to the demands of children or partner, your body will most certainly not have had what it needs for continued healthy functioning.

You Are the Most Powerful Authority on Your Own Well-being

The effect of your lifestyle on your body and your emotions is direct and profound. This system of medicine, reflexology, takes into account every aspect of your life and can help you address any problems you may have, allowing you to make sense of the whole rather than covering up or stopping the effects of a difficult day. Simply covering up the effects will not enable you to heal and improve your well-being.

As your emotions have an effect on the workings of your body so does the functioning of your body affect the flow of your emotions. For instance, the liver regulates digestive activity — it makes bile (stored in the gall bladder), which deals with fats; it stores and filters blood; and it controls the emotions. A healthy liver will help to maintain healthy emotions that may be spontaneously felt, expressed, and released, allowing you to move on to the next event. On the other hand, a troubled liver with impaired functioning will be unable to do this and may aggravate emotional turbulence. Just how the reduced functioning of the liver affects you as a whole is complex and far-reaching; how the problems may be understood and repaired is clearly shown in meridian theory.

How Reflexology Can Help You

If you choose to use reflexology you will receive treatment that takes into account and enhances your whole person: the way your body works, which in turn affects the way your mind is able to work; and your lifestyle and the stresses you are under, which affect the emotions you feel and how they flow. To take one of these aspects of your life and treat it in isolation without regard for the influence that it has on the whole leads to a series of problems, each arising out of the last, due to never taking action appropriate to the whole picture. Actions arising from decisions taken without sufficient information generally prove to be less than satisfactory — incomplete at best, and causing further problems at worst.

Natural Laws

The earth and all that lives and has its being on it has certain natural laws that govern how things work. If we go against these laws we ourselves may suffer, or cause suffering, but we cannot change the pattern — the blueprint — of how things work. For example, you cannot make water flow uphill (you can push it but it will never naturally flow that way); you cannot make apples fall upward because the laws of gravity cannot be contravened. That's how the world works whether we like it or not.

You cannot make water stay in one place and not move, except by containing it behind a dam — but that is the action of the dam not the water because water continues to behave as it always has and will. In fact, you cannot make anything stay the same because natural law dictates that *life is a state of change*. Everything that is alive is constantly changing — if it wasn't it would be dead. We now know that we are composed of atoms that are constantly moving and replacing themselves. Therefore I am not composed today of one single particle of that matter that was me seven years ago, yet each particle conforms to the blueprint that is me. Likewise the blueprint that is the natural law of the universe shapes the way that life on the earth works.

Saint Augustine said that there are no miracles, only ignorance of natural laws. The earth has a built-in blueprint or program that works superbly, always to the best advantage of living things. When we go against that law so we are fighting life itself and we will be less alive and will suffer.

We Are Made of the Food We Eat

Even when creatures or plants are themselves dead, they are part of life and change gradually to become the earth that is the goodness that sustains life as we know it. None of us would be alive without the earth to grow our food. Food plays a major part in our health today (as it always has, of course) and is something we overlook at our peril. Your car will not run without gasoline; you will not run without the fuel, which is food, to make your body function. *If you do not feed your body you will die, therefore what you are is the food you eat — you are made of what you eat.* What happens if you put the wrong kind of gasoline in your car, if you put diesel into a gasoline engine by mistake? It will not function at all. If you put in the wrong octane gasoline the car will become "ill" — it will not run well, it will cough, and splutter.

What Is Good Food?

The quality of the food you eat will have a direct and profound effect on your health. Food that is grown in a natural, organic way will be rich in the enzymes that your body needs; whereas the more food is interfered with in the growing process, the less it can supply your essential needs. Chemical additives to the soil (fertilizers) and to the plant to help it grow (pesticides and hormones) change the essential nature of the organism and make it poorer in goodness, which means poorer in the natural substances you need for your body's healthy functioning. The more foodstuffs are processed the more quality is lost from that food. The balance of nutrients will be interfered with to such a degree that the food may become unstable. For example, butter is now thought to be better for you than processed sunflower margarine because it has been shown that the highly valued polyunsaturates are so changed in processing that they actually become a highly unstable saturated fat.

Fruit that ripens naturally on the plant is alkaline in nature, whereas fruit that has been picked green and changes color after transportation, at the point of supply by exposure to certain gasses is highly acidic. These fruits are not ripened by the gasses — they never ripen, but just become unripe fruit that *looks* ripe. In effect they are dead fruit because they are arrested at the point of picking and do not develop.

Have you ever bought pears that seem hard and you expect to ripen in the warmth of your home only to find that they go from unripe to rotten (from the center outward)? This is not living but dead food: it is going against the laws of nature, which mandate that food ripens from the green state and progresses to ripe, then to overripe and then decays. These unripened fruits die at the point of picking just as a premature baby will die if it is born much too early. They also, incidentally, lack many of the essential nutrients that we expect to find in fruit: "fruit is good for you" may be less than true these days, unless you grow your own or select naturally produced, organically grown food.

We Eat Too Much and Yet Are Suffering from Malnutrition

The majority of people today are suffering from a form of starvation because their bodies are just not getting what they need in the form of essential nutrients to function efficiently. They cannot get what they need from the partly artificial food that is normally available. Is it not bizarre, or tragic, that we have to go out of our way to find food that is nourishing, that we are surrounded by an abundance that is actually not good for us? It is like magic food in a children's fairy tale that looks wonderfully formed and perfect yet is actually "bad."

We Are Slowly Poisoning Ourselves

Most of us are also suffering to some extent from poisoning, both from the additives in our food (polluted food) and from the polluted air we breathe. We are also suffering from toxins manufactured within our own bodies as a response to malfunctioning (as a result of what we have looked at above). Toxins are produced by negative emotions and the stresses of living a "modern" life in bodies that were designed for life thousands of years ago. We do not always notice the effects of this toxicity but wonder why we catch so many bugs and do not feel in good health, or wonder why we feel so lacking in energy and vitality that life always seems difficult.

People Are One of the Greatest Achievements of Creation

Our bodies have, as yet, evolved very little to adapt to a life dictated and shaped by technology and "scientific" developments. We can fly to the moon but we still put food in one end and the waste products come out the other! And that is not to say that we are in any way primitive. The intricate processes that sustain life in our body are unimaginably complex and subtly balanced. They put the technology of space travel to shame by their complexity. So also are the powers of our mind and its potential. Most people use only a small fraction of their mental potential and intuitive abilities. What most effectively inhibits this terrific potential? It is the effect of the all to frequent negative emotions, of the distress we all feel from our early life onward.

How Distress Affects Us

The pattern of distress clouding our mental functioning and working detrimentally on our bodily processes starts from conception, though, of course, we cannot keep track of it. An example of this is a baby in the first three months after birth who may feel hungry while the mother is unavailable or unwilling to feed it yet. The baby feels hungry, creating a "wanting" feeling in its tummy, a need, something missing. This is expressed as pain because what is not right feels wrong and a need that is not supplied causes pain. The baby will not comprehend that mother and food are coming — it has not yet developed the conscious faculties to think beyond the moment — and the feeling it is experiencing, which is hunger. With no way of knowing whether this need will ever be supplied again the pain stretches into infinity for the baby.

This baby will not be able to recall the experience consciously, but the feeling of hunger pain coupled with despair will remain in the body all its life to be recognized as distress if circumstances should cause the body to tense up and feel discomfort in the same areas again. We all carry within our bodies our own set of weaknesses that we respond to based on traumas and shocks we have experienced. The things that undermine our strength might flow off someone else "like water off a duck's back" because they do not have an early experience of the thing as trauma, outside their control. Yet something that we take in stride might well cause distress and problems to another person.

STRESS IS NATURAL — DISTRESS IS ILLNESS

Stress is a natural part of life: without stress your body would collapse in a useless heap on the ground. It is the balance between the muscles holding the structures together in a state of some stress that keeps us upright (that is how bridges and buildings work). It is stress in the form of challenge that stimulates our minds to grow and develop. But excessive stress becomes dis-stress, which is trouble.

The reflexologist practicing in a holistic way comes into all this when distress has upset the balance of our being. All a reflexologist (or other holistic practitioner) can do is to help redress the balance. This is no mean achievement because it is the balance of body, mind, and spirit within our bodies that is the essence of health in its fullest sense. How this balance is achieved is what *Discover Reflexology* is about.

WHAT IS REFLEXOLOGY?

You may ask: "How can it be that a therapy that works only on the feet (or hands) can claim to affect the whole body? Surely if I have something wrong with my feet I might visit a reflexologist, but how could she/he help with my asthma or irritable bowel syndrome?"

That it does help is illustrated by the number of people who leave their reflexologist after a course of treatment experiencing permanent relief from the problems that caused them to seek help in the first place. Reflexology can provide relief because the whole body is represented on the feet and hands through points that can be individually stimulated to produce a reaction in the corresponding body part. If I am having a consultation with someone who has a stiff and painful left shoulder following a sports injury it is not unusual for them to remark as I work the corresponding part on the foot that they feel a sensation of immediate relief in their shoulder.

THE FLOW OF ENERGY AROUND THE BODY

How can there be a link between the two parts? This happens because the body is linked by energy flowing along certain pathways. When stimulation is applied on one point along the line it will travel along and around that line until it has traveled through every part of the body that lies in its pathway. When an impulse travels along a line it will stimulate everything that lies in its path. Organs and body parts that are functioning well will allow energy to flow through freely with little change. When the impulse meets a damaged area, however, the physiological effect of the increased flow of energy will be to stimulate that part to heal itself.

Imagine a stream traveling along its path. Where it is clear the stream will run along freely, covering the miles effortlessly. But if it should meet boulders in its path, or a fallen tree, the water will be restricted and will push and squeeze its way through the constricted area. It will work gradually to clear the path of congestion so that it can proceed more fully. Or, imagine an electrical circuit. Energy will always keep flowing, it will pass through things — or around things if they do not conduct electricity — but it cannot stop and disappear. Just as your blood travels around your body and flows without ceasing while you are alive, so electromagnetic energy flows constantly through our bodies.

This has not yet been fully explained or understood in relation to the human body, yet it is a clearly explained and central part of physics. (Physics is the study of natural science and particularly of the properties — other than chemical — of matter and energy.) We are part of the natural world and are indisputably composed of matter and energy. Therefore it seems probable that we will soon understand energy much more fully. Indeed, research has and is being carried out that has already increased our understanding of these matters. In 1628, when it was first suggested by William Harvey that the blood circulated around our bodies, the idea was received incredulously and the theory treated as heretical. We seem to be going through much the same process today with regard to the energy in our bodies.

Why Reflex Points? What Is a Reflex?

Most of us are familiar with the knee-jerk reflex that doctors use to test our reactions. This involves a circuit in the nervous system that travels to the spinal cord and back without involving the brain. The reflexes on the feet do not work through this very simple process. It has not yet been fully explained what the reflexes of reflexology are (they are linked with the flow of energy around the body and will no doubt be better understood when both are further researched), but we do know how the reflexes work. We know that pressure applied to the foot produces a mirrored response in the body and that the response will be found in specific parts according to the specific points of the foot that have been touched. The link between these corresponding parts seems to be through energy rather than through a direct material link.

Therapy Given with the Hands

Treatment is given with the hands using pressure techniques: the fingers applying specific pressure to areas that are sometimes very small points. A reflexology treatment consists of stimulation to specific points given within a foot massage. Reflexology is not foot massage, which is a relaxing, whole-hand massage technique applied to the feet to stimulate and generally relax the body. Reflexology uses foot massage to prepare and relax the feet for specific pressure techniques that are precisely aimed to correspond to individual organs or body parts.

The Body Is Mirrored on the Feet

You can see from Illustration 1 how the side view of the human form corresponds closely to the side view of the foot. The curves of the spine are exactly mirrored in the curves around the bony structure of the foot.

Now look at Illustration 2 and see how the two feet together roughly represent the human torso. The spine runs down the center of the instep of each foot where the center of the body lies. The head and neck are represented on the toes and the neck of the toes: the big toe represents the whole head, with fine tuning for the eyes, ears, neck, and teeth found on the smaller toes. The ball of the foot is the chest area bounded by the diaphragm. The abdomen lies in the instep and the pelvic area is all around the heel.

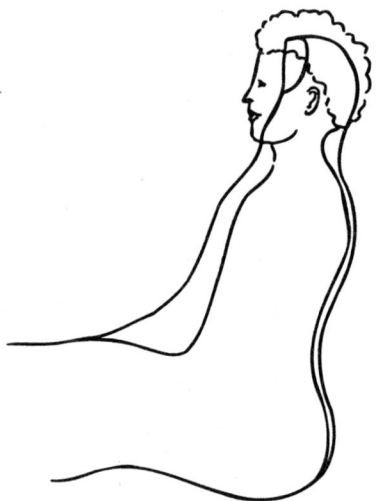

Illustration 1
Side View of the Foot Compared to the Human Form

You may notice that the limbs do not feature much on the feet, although the charts will show you where to work for the shoulder, arm, knee, and leg. The limbs are superimposed on to other areas. When you have a specific problem on a limb, for instance tennis elbow, you would work the

Illustration 2
How the Body Fits on to the Feet

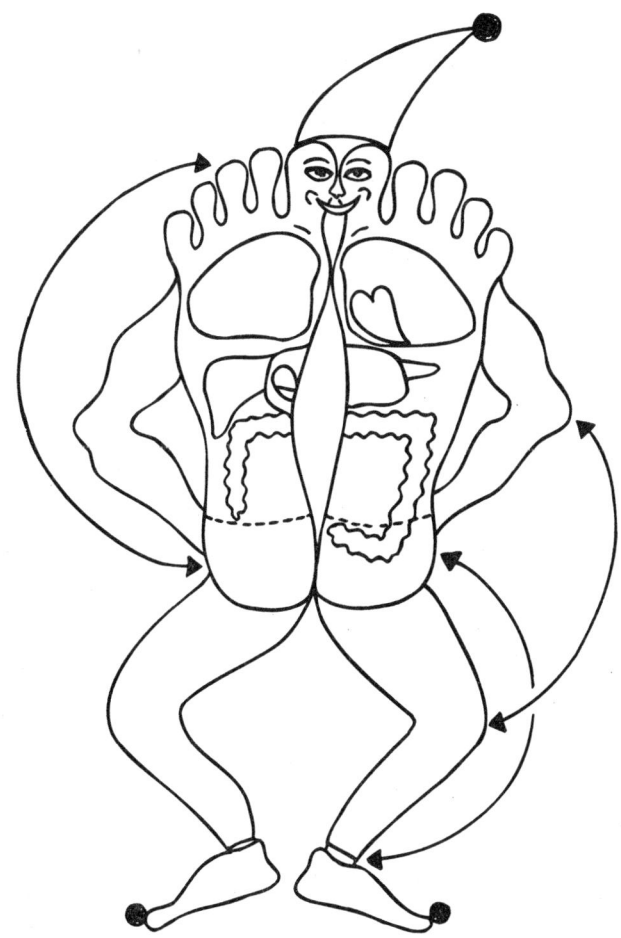

Shoulder corresponds with hip, hip with shoulder
Elbow corresponds with knee, knee with elbow
Wrist corresponds with ankle, ankle with wrist
Cross reflexes correspond to the corresponding part
  on the same side of the body, both ways

arm area on the foot, but you would also work that area on the matching limb. Therefore for someone with tennis elbow in their right arm you would work the corresponding joint on the right leg, which is the knee (see Illustration 2). These reflexes found on the limbs are referred to as cross reflexes (working across from one limb to the other on the same side).

In this way, all the various parts of the body fit onto the feet — the left and right feet mirroring the left and right sides of the body. Wherever there is illness in the body we can find a corresponding area in the foot that may be tender or painful, and where waste materials have collected in the form of deposits. Reflexology works by massaging the feet to break down these deposits, dispersing the pain, and restoring the energy flow to a state of balance. Tension is relaxed throughout the muscles and the nervous system, and circulation is increased, releasing or reducing the strain from which the body is suffering.

How Reflexology Affects the Body

When the energy is flowing freely around your body you are physically, mentally, and emotionally well, balanced, and in harmony with your environment. The functioning of the organs is improved by releasing tension held in the body. Muscles control the workings of the organs (each tiny hair on your skin has its own muscles, for example, and your digestive system can only function through its own set of muscles) as well as large movements of the body through activity of the limbs. Treatment stimulates the circulation of the blood and lymph so that the removal of waste products and toxins is increased and the supply of nutrients throughout the blood supply is improved. By releasing long-term muscular contractions the constrictions they have imposed on the nerves are relieved and the nerve supply is freed. These are the physiological effects of reflexology treatment.

What Does It Feel Like?

Patients receiving reflexology treatment often feel tenderness as certain points are worked, and they usually experience an immediate release of tensions (some will experience an initial reaction or healing crisis). This can be seen as well as felt when a person who comes in tired and depleted changes their whole attitude with the relaxing of tension. A glow of vitality can be seen as the energy flow begins to restore balance and well-being.

The number of treatments needed vary according to the type of disorder and the length of time it has been suffered. Usually the trouble yields more quickly when it is of recent origin. When a great deal of repair and healing is needed the time required for recovery is longer.

Reflexology is an ideal way of treating children. They invariably enjoy it and it is non-invasive (therefore not threatening). It is also very effective. But the pressure used must be much lighter than for adults. Babies, too, can be treated by an experienced reflexologist who knows how to adapt the pressure: for a very young baby just a few weeks old it is sufficient to stroke gently the points on the feet with one finger. The results will be immediately apparent.

THE HISTORY OF REFLEXOLOGY

In some parts of the world reflexology is a fully accredited medical treatment. It is often used as an accurate form of diagnosis, foretelling disturbances in the body long before they become physically apparent. It is also used to correct imbalances before they become serious.

HEALING IN ANCIENT CIVILIZATIONS

Foot treatment was widely practiced in China, Egypt, and India thousands of years ago. The earliest known record of working the feet is found on a wall painting in an Egyptian pyramid, known as the physician's tomb, dating to about 2330 B.C. It shows two physicians treating two wealthy patients, one working on the feet, and the other the hands. North American Indians have a tradition of foot massage. Central to their philosophy is the understanding that the feet are our connection with the Earth and the Universe.

Reflexology is based on the ancient Chinese understanding of health and the flow of energy around the body. Ancient Chinese medical care was based on the understanding of man as a whole being, not just as a collection of parts. If illness occurred it was recognized as a problem of the whole being because body and mind were seen to be totally interrelated. The ancient Chinese believed that the connecting link throughout is energy, the life force known as *Ch'i*, which connects our being into a living whole.

Illness was seen to be an imbalance, or congestion, in the body restricting the passage of this energy. The aim of medical care was to free the constrictions and balance the energy flow so that the illness could be healed by the freely flowing energy. It is this energy that maintains our health. Every part of the body was shown to be on one of the various pathways, or meridians, of energy so that an inner organ could be reached by working on points along the pathway related to it. Further, every organ and part of the body was seen to have reflex points (that is points that correspond to the organ through energy) in other parts of the body. Some of the most sensitive of these are found in the feet and hands. Acupuncture uses needles to stimulate the points on the energy lines, shiatsu uses pressure. Reflexology uses pressure applied with the hands that concentrates almost entirely on the feet.

In ancient China reflexology and acupuncture were practiced together. Reflexology was used to locate imbalances or problems and to treat the whole body; needles were then applied on specific meridian points. During that time there were two forms of acupuncture. The rich man's physician practiced what is known as Five Element acupuncture and treated the whole person — body, mind, emotions, and spirit. He applied his needles singly to points called spirit points, for the well-being of the whole. He was only paid while the patient remained well. The poor received treatment for their ailments from the Barefoot Doctor who walked from village to village with his needles. He would apply many needles at once to relieve the symptoms that his patients experienced. This is the type of acupuncture you are more likely to receive today, unless your practitioner practices Traditional Chinese acupuncture (Five Element acupuncture). Traditional Chinese medicine commonly uses many needles at once, together with herbal preparations and other treatments.

Developments in Europe and the West

From the fourteenth century onward pressure point therapy was used in Europe in one form or another. The development of reflexology, however, primarily came about in the latter part of the last century by doctors who were unaware of meridian theory. The main interest was in Germany and the United States where Dr. William Fitzgerald, among others, produced a simplified form of the theory of energy pathways—zone therapy—that he used for analgesic and anesthetizing effects. His interest and enthusiasm played a major role in spreading the knowledge of this therapy in the Western world. During that time reflexology was being developed in the West independently of the knowledge and practice of pressure therapy and meridian theory in other parts of the world.

Eunice Ingham was the founder of reflexology as we know it today. She was the first to realize the full benefits of the therapy as expounded by Dr. Fitzgerald. She concentrated mainly on the feet, making a detailed map of the reflexes found there. She also used pressure therapy to relieve congestion and stimulate the healing processes, whereas zone therapy had previously been used mainly for numbing body parts to give pain relief. Her work has been continued throughout the world by many people, particularly her nephew, Dwight Byers.

Recent Progress

In the 1960s, Robert St. John was working mainly on the spinal reflex area of the feet. He developed the Metamorphic Technique, or Metamorphosis, from his basic work in reflexology. Robert St. John's attention was drawn to observing and learning about the psychological effects of treatment, especially the effects he found from working the spine. The spine is the main bony support for the whole body and contains part of the central nervous system. Because body and mind are fully interrelated this appeared to be a key area for treatment.

Reflexology, with the understanding that Metamorphosis has brought to it, releases the healing forces latent in the body and enables the life force (energy) to bring about change within the patient. Changes may manifest themselves on the mental and emotional levels as well as on the physical level.

Currently, Inge Dougans is at the forefront of bringing the knowledge of East and West together by showing that the zones of reflexology are probably a simplified form of identifying the energy pathways, which are more thoroughly plotted as the meridians of acupuncture.

4

HOW REFLEXOLOGY WORKS

Our feet are at the end of the line, bearing all our weight, and are often neglected and frequently mistreated. We squeeze them into ill-fitting shoes that are a different shape from our feet. We wash them when we bath or shower, but often do not really look at them. They become dry with peeling or hard, cracked skin, or develop unchecked fungal or viral infections, such as athlete's foot or verrucas. Yet the feet are surprisingly responsive and sensitive when attended to or stimulated. It is common for people to not feel a great deal during their first reflexology treatment, but over a few sessions they are amazed to find just how much feeling they have in their feet. Others find that they experience a lot of tenderness and feeling in their feet from the start. They are often intrigued by the connections with sensations in other parts of their body.

If somebody wants to receive reflexology it may be that they would like to have some time and nurturing for themselves, or they may have a health problem they want help with.

What Happens in a Reflexology Treatment

A reflexology treatment starts by comfortably positioning the person receiving treatment so that their feet are raised and their legs are supported. Some questions need to be asked to ascertain whether there is any serious illness or trouble that should be taken into account. If you visit a reflexology practitioner this will take the form of a consultation during which the practitioner takes a relevant medical history as well as asks about the reasons for coming and how you are feeling.

Initial contact will then be made with the hands on your feet, with gentle massage to warm and prepare them, and some vigorous massage movements to stimulate the circulation. Treatment usually lasts for up to an hour. During this time you will receive a lot of foot massage and within this the various reflex points will be stimulated, using pressure techniques. Sometimes treatment will take longer when trouble is encountered, or on a large pair of feet. On the other hand, children's feet are smaller than adults' and they would not benefit from prolonged treatment because their metabolism is faster and their attention span shorter. Elderly people may be fragile and might not need a treatment that is as long or uses as much pressure as a middle-aged adult.

The benefits of reflexology include a feeling of relaxation as treatment progresses, with a sense of well-being by completion of the session. Some people will experience a passing sensation of tenderness or discomfort as pressure is applied to a particular point where there is congestion but this will be followed by a feeling of ease or of increased warmth.

During treatment there is a relaxation of contracted muscles so that the surrounding areas of the body are freed from constriction. Thus the nerve supply is not compressed and can work freely; the circulation and glands are stimulated; and energy is able to flow more freely around the body. Stimulation of the circulation has several important results: the supply of oxygen and nutrients to all parts of the body is increased and toxins and waste products are efficiently carried away by the lymph and blood, enabling the whole body to function better. The patient may feel relaxed or energized according to "what is going on for them." Energy will be able to flow around their body more freely, enhancing all the physical and emotional processes.

SELF-HEALING

Reflexology allows the self-healing processes to take place. The reflexologist could be said to serve as the body's housecleaner — promoting removal of the waste products that are inhibiting the free functioning of the body systems. Once the garbage has been cleared the body naturally functions more fully and self-healing takes over. Practitioners do not heal anything: they only remove the impediments or the barriers to healing so that the individual mind/body/spirit can make its own choices.

As a practitioner my intention is to offer my expertise and awareness in the manner of an open door through which the individual patient may look and choose to go or not. Each person is the best authority on what is right for them when they are able to see the choices available.

THE EFFECTS OF TREATMENT

Treatment works on the physical and mental levels, relieving muscles that have become tense in response to hurt feelings (emotional) or physical hurt. It gives the body/mind/spirit a chance to release tensions that are inhibiting free functioning and health. All physical complaints and disease are a result of a reaction to some trauma: sometimes initially physical (as in an accident), sometimes emotional, but always having an emotional/mental element (how we feel about what happened). In the case of an accident the question may arise: was the person perhaps temporarily distracted from taking care and if so what had occurred to cause this? Any kind of trauma is recorded in the body as muscular tension in the body parts and organs affected.

Reflexology treatment loosens these tensions and traumas both physically and mentally, touching the root cause of the disease. This gives the patient an opportunity to release the tensions and recover from their lasting effects. Where traumas are of recent or incipient origin the release of the tension involved acts in a preventative way, resolving the imbalance before it can adversely affect the body in any long-term manner.

The practitioner works alongside the patient, offering expertise in health and general well-being. However, she knows better than the patient about individual timing and choices.

How Often?

How often treatment should be given depends largely on the individual. It is crucial that the person receiving treatment has time to assimilate the effects and find a new equilibrium. Frequency of treatment should match the individual's own pace. On the other hand, where a disease is deep-seated and of long duration treatment will need to be given often enough to help the organism bring about some change or the body will revert to old habits between sessions. As a general rule, a course of treatment for a specific condition reflects the length of time the condition has been present; where the problem is of recent origin results may be expected sooner than in a long-established illness.

WHAT DO WE MEAN BY HEALTH?

It is worthwhile considering what we mean by health. Is health an absence of illness? Are we healthy if we are not suffering from any illness that seriously restricts us? Or is the state of health something positive: a feeling of physical and emotional well-being and clear mental functioning? If you know a doctor, ask them to define health and see if you agree. *The American Heritage Dictionary* states that health is a condition of wholesomeness or soundness of body or mind.

DIS-EASE

Disease is really dis-ease, a lack of ease or well-being. It is defined in the dictionary as uneasiness, a disorder or want of health in mind or body, a cause of pain.

Any dis-ease gets in the way of our well-being and the healthy functioning of our body. Without dis-ease our well-being is maintained by the life force of the body/person. Health is a natural state and one which we always strive to get back to even on a level we are not aware of; it is absolutely built-in. Self-healing takes place as a result of the life force within the living thing, be it plant or animal.

Life Is a State of Change

You can last for about three minutes without breathing. You can live for about three days without water and for about three weeks without food. Air, water, and food are essential for life. Life is always in a state of change; nothing that is living remains set in the same condition. Our matter is composed of atoms that are constantly on the move; our cells renew; our skin and hair drop off and are replaced. Stagnation and lack of mobility inhibits life—restricts and eventually throttles it as it prevents renewal. Health, therefore, requires a state of flexibility both in body and mind. This is ease. Tightness does not have ease of movement. Every emotion has its own physical manifestation: it is not possible to feel something without experiencing the effect of that feeling within your body. We usually overlook this in our daily lives.

The freedom of movement in the body of the muscles (and therefore of the circulation and nervous system) will enable them to function to their potential — this is a state of health. This should be the natural state of functioning in all of us. When we experience trouble our bodies should restore us to this state automatically as the problem passes. What happens more often is that troubles accumulate and the problems they cause accumulate correspondingly. Our self-healing processes then become overloaded and out of balance and we do not get well without help. Reflexology acts exactly as the self-healing process works. Indeed what it does is activate self-healing.

Flexibility of response enables you to have the appropriate reactions to challenging situations. This is the healthy way to live. Emotions that are flowing freely, with understanding of how you are feeling, will not restrict you and trap you in a set way of responding. When you can look at what is in front of you and see it for what it is you can make appropriate decisions. However, when you have a fearful, rigid, and defensive reaction to a pile of old emotions attached to feelings you are experiencing on a particular occasion (or moment) you may have a certain constriction of choice—you narrow this new experience by trying it to fit into the memory you have of the last time you felt this way.

When you are able to approach a problem in the moment, without old baggage, you will be able to find creative solutions rather than be trapped by habitual responses based on old memories. This is not something you can do using willpower. It happens naturally when you let yourself become aware of how you are feeling, when you try to listen to what your feelings and body are telling you about what you have just experienced. Often this does not match what you are thinking about a situation, but it will become an increasingly helpful and an accurate guide to how and who you really are (rather than what you would like to think you are).

Lack of Change Leads to Stagnation

So, if the state of being alive is a state of change, then to be less alive than your potential is to be in a state of reduced movement or stagnation. This is commonly referred to as a blockage in energy flow. This is inaccurate, however, as blockage would result in death; what is meant is partial blockage — constriction.

Change Is Scary

One way in which the necessity for change manifests itself is in our attitudes. If you try changing your attitude you will find that you get more from what you focus on. For instance, if you spend all day worrying about where your son has lost his wallet you will probably have an anxious day. On the other hand, you may look for it and then say to yourself you have done the best you can and there is no more that you can do at present. You may then decide to do other things with your day and put your trust in the universe to produce the wallet if it is going to be found. In this way you also acknowledge that it is your son's wallet and it is his responsibility although you would have liked to help him if you could. The chances are the wallet will be found when an idea pops into someone's mind and is acted upon. A tight and anxious mind does not open to such casual thoughts or coincidences because it is too rigid in its focus.

Test this theory in other ways. People who are rigidly anxious about a forthcoming exam will often be unable to do as well as they could if their mind/body are relaxed and open, able to let thought flow freely through it. People who are able to focus on doing well in an exam are usually those who can handle the process relatively well and achieve good results: their mind and body are able to function freely and adapt to need. If you are having money problems it is easy to become locked in a poverty trap. Yet some people have the experience of suddenly receiving funding when they need it, apparently out of the blue, by believing the need and trust will be provided from somewhere. One person will survive and recover from a terrible accident whereas another will not.

What you believe, what you hold in your mind, is of crucial importance in shaping your life. We develop and use our bodies, we develop and use our brains, and we can develop and use our consciousness if we desire. If we do not will it, life will often push us into situations where we have the opportunity, or are forced, to have another go around.

Getting to Know Yourself

If you feel upset about something try this experiment. First take the time to notice how you feel and recognize what has made you feel upset and why it upset you. When you have felt the relief of acknowledging what is "bugging" you it is like a light going on: "Oh! That is what really troubled me!" Then put into your mind what you would like for yourself and keep remembering and restating it. If you think you know what was troubling you but still feel confused you probably haven't gotten to the bottom of it: how you actually feel. See which approach is most likely to bring about a satisfactory change: focusing on the problem and letting yourself become immersed in it, or envisaging what would work and be good for you and getting a feel for that.

Experts in Good Health or Ill Health?

Medical training makes a study of ill health. Doctors are experts in diagnosing disease and in knowing the options for treatment of advanced diseases where self-help alone may not be enough to change an established condition. Practitioners of complementary or alternative medicine have chiefly studied well-being. Their expertise lies in helping people find out for themselves what they feel is wrong. Alternative medicine practitioners enable people to find out what they can do to help themselves, how they can liberate themselves by feeling empowered to make changes, to take charge of their own lives.

Imagine introducing the ancient Chinese system of only paying your practitioner while you remain well (because if you become sick they are not doing their job of enabling you to remain healthy). That would give *health* care a very clear focus as health care. It would protect against the tendency to pay isolated attention to a local problem, out of its context as part of the whole body (and out of the context of the body as part of the totality of our being: body/mind/spirit).

Recognizing and Naming Problems

A responsible complementary practitioner will never diagnose a named medical condition or medically name a trouble, but will refer a client to his doctor to identify the problem. Once this has been done it is up to each individual to choose the treatment they feel is right for them. You are under no obligation to accept treatment that you do not want from anyone at all. Some people find that invasive treatment leads to further invasive treatment as a result of complications; others recognize a need for drastic immediate action in their particular case. The important thing for each of us to remember is that each individual has her own unique experience of an illness; where two people have a disease that carries the same name there will always be as much personal variation to take into account as there will be common factors.

Reflexology shows up in areas of constriction or congestion long before there is a named illness. It highlights areas of trouble. Perhaps you have had a difficult week at work and feel pressured and uptight. This tightness will be felt in your body and it is this tension that the reflexology treatment will work on to release so you can function more fully again. When people labor for years under excessive stress their bodies may become damaged from the prolonged inhibition of the bodily processes. It is then that you may get a named condition.

Disease Does Not Strike "Out of the Blue"

Disease is the tip of the iceberg: most of an iceberg lies under the water and only one twentieth shows visibly above. Disease builds up unseen and unnoticed over months and years. Often it is only when it is serious enough to be a named condition that we start to do something serious about it. Doctors are so overloaded in dealing with patients with specified disease that they do not have much time to attend to those whose troubles are not yet serious enough to manifest themselves as a named condition.

It is a common experience to visit a general practitioner and be told (to your relief) that there is "nothing wrong." How often is this relief replaced with a vague disquiet? "If there is nothing wrong then why am I feeling so terrible? Or, "Why am I experiencing this continued discomfort?" The answer is that something is wrong but it is not yet a named disease. If we are able to do something to change the cause of that discomfort, that is to make a change in the contributing factors creating that discomfort, then we will be able to relieve ourselves (mind and body) of the cause of illness before it becomes serious.

MAKING CHANGES TO HEAL OURSELVES

This can be brought about by anything. It may be that a coincidence will show us a way to change things, or we may consult a complementary practitioner who may be able to help us recognize the issues and find our own strength (physical and emotional) to make the changes necessary for our own health. If we visit a practitioner who we do not feel is quite right for us, or if we receive treatment that is not having any effect, then it is important to consider whether this is perhaps not the appropriate person for us at this time.

The individual practitioner will have as much effect on the outcome of treatment as will the specific discipline, if not more. Reflexology, for example, may or may not be the best treatment to begin to shift the condition that has been troubling you and help to bring about changes in your illness. (However, I personally believe that it can be of potential, though not necessarily exclusive, benefit in every case.) It may be that it would seem too slow a process initially and that another therapy, such as homeopathy, might just "kick start" the healing process. It might equally be that the particular reflexologist you visited was not the "right" person for you at that particular time.

TRAUMA AND DISEASE

If health is a state of ease or well-being that we slip from when under excessive stress from pressure or trauma then it is useful to be aware of the physical effects of pressure and trauma.

Try this for yourself. During the day notice when you feel uncomfortable. This is not as easy as it sounds. Most of us are so accustomed to feeling uneasy a lot of the time that we do not readily notice when we are in that state. But it is possible with awareness. So when you notice that you are feeling uncomfortable make a note of where in your body you feel tightness, or pain, or sickness. Then think back over the past few minutes or hours of the day and what has happened. As you run through events or conversations you will probably recognize what it was that made you uneasy. Do not discount something because it seems small or unimportant—these things can set off feelings in us that are quite powerful, even if we don't know why. This will often be because the apparently little thing reminds us of an earlier (maybe years earlier and maybe recurring) situation in which we have been made to feel acutely uneasy or hurt or scared. Though we may not even recognize the similarity or identify the memory, it will trigger in us a similarly uneasy response or reaction.

Do Problems "Get You Going?"

It is not usually possible to change your situation in life overnight, though it can be. What each one of us can do to help ourselves is to notice how the little stresses exacerbate our troubles, or how our way of reacting to recurring problems makes our life more difficult, more stressful.

For example, if one of my children is unhappy and needing some help when it is time for me to leave for the clinic I have to make a choice between attending to my child and arriving on time. What I will probably do will be to spend just enough time to enable my child to cope, by acknowledging his feelings or showing him that someone else can help.

I will then leave, short of time, and while I drive to the clinic I will feel anxious that my client may arrive early and be waiting, puzzled, on the doorstep. I now know from experience that my choice here is between a natural anxiety or a willed compassion for myself as having done the best I can. It is not actually too difficult to apologize to someone and explain that my child was distressed and that was why I was held up.

I know that if I can believe that I have done the best I possibly can, instead of abandoning my child (temporarily), or expecting the impossible of myself by trying to be in two places at once, I will give a better treatment and so actually serve my client well. Whereas if I crush myself with anxiety (guilt), for something that I chose to do because it was important, I will be doubly failing the other person both by keeping them waiting and then not giving of my best during treatment. But if from my life experience I am anxious that my client will be hostile and that I will be severely criticized or verbally attacked and I am shrinking (quite naturally) from that psychic attack, this will be a difficult thing to do. However much sense it may make to me in my mind I will not be able to *feel* that sense in my body, where the overriding feeling will be one of anxiety about the forthcoming attack. Only compassion for myself, that I have ever been made to feel like this, will probably enable me to override my pattern of reaction and find the strength to go through with what makes sense.

How We Really Are or Who We Like to Think We Are

This is why New Year's resolutions can be so demoralizing: We recognize where we go "wrong" and understand how we would like to be, but intending to do "better" does not in any way change how we feel. However much you impose your will upon yourself sooner or later your feelings will break out in some way. Only if you can have compassion and recognition for how you *actually feel* and understand just how difficult the task is that you have set yourself (even if it seems intellectually quite possible) will you have a chance of success.

You Cannot Change Anyone Except Yourself

We cannot change other people, but we can change ourselves. We can change our responses if we wish and if we can find compassion for ourselves and what we are suffering. This is much harder to do than to say because most of us are used to having to "get on with it" — to put up with things. But if we cannot have compassion for ourselves in our own suffering who else is going to?

Disease is Dis-ease or Distress

It is crucial that we come to take very seriously indeed the fact that disease is a result of dis-ease, that illness comes about when the person suffering it can find no relief from the strain they are experiencing in mind or body. Whether the body has been attacked by a virulent virus or by great stress and pressure in the person's life, the cause will gradually wear it down until the body says "no more" and throws out some kind of reaction to the excessive load it finds itself under. We are all familiar with the infectious disease that passes some people by, sparing them while prostrating many around them. Or we feel caught unaware when we catch the flu because we "never have the flu" — we haven't had it for years although it has been so prevalent around us. Whatever the reaction, our body will find some way to protest if it is laboring under too much strain.

It would be a much better explanation and expression of the process to say "I have illness" rather than "I am ill." After all, we do say "I have a headache" or "I have the flu," so why not "I have illness?" What I *am* is a whole person with unlimited potential — we all are. If I experience or have illness it is because something is not right — my body/mind/spirit is unable to continue in a state of well-being and so it is sounding warning signals. I know that I do not catch infectious diseases unless I am already weakened by something. Normally I do not worry about visiting or touching someone who is suffering from an infection of some kind because if I am all right I do not catch things. If I am tired or vulnerable for some reason, however, then I am more likely to be susceptible.

You Are Your Own Healer — The Experts Are Merely Your Assistants

All healing is self-healing, a result of the inner healing process or life force. We may need help in some form or another, but when we have received that help we will only get better if we make use of it.

The common cold is the result of a virus we have picked up and our body will gather all the strengths of its immune system to combat the infection. The white blood cells will increase (more will be made) and they will act to kill the invading forces and to clear the toxins from our body. Our noses stream as our respiratory system works overtime to clear the toxins out by making large quantities of mucus as the means to carry them away. If we care for ourselves and rest when we need to and can the cold will be over and done with in a few days with no outside intervention.

Ask any doctor or surgeon about "the will to live," which will show itself in patients with life-threatening diseases who make "miraculous" recoveries against the odds. When two people have had pneumonia, or the same serious operation, their recovery will not be the same. It will be in accordance with their will to live, the strength of their life force or capacity for self-healing. It is crucial that we realize that it is up to us how we are.

When we are in trouble we may be able to work through it ourselves or we may need help. If we need help we may go to a friend or someone we can trust; we may go to the doctor for medication to deaden the pain; or we may go to another kind of practitioner seeking help to strengthen our self-healing. But if we want to be well we have to find some way — on our own or with help—of enabling our self-healing processes.

Victim or Boss?

When an illness hits you from out of the blue you can regard it as an external force that has taken you over and go to the doctor or pharmacist for some "magic" medicine to take it away. Or, you can stop and look at yourself and feel the pain or discomfort, looking back to see what has caused you to feel uneasy or hurt prior to succumbing to the pain. If you understand that your well-being is a result of the functioning of your own inner healing process it can be wonderfully liberating: "I am really in charge! I can shape how things go for me." You may need help but you are the boss. On the other hand, it can be absolutely terrifying: "I am responsible for everything that happens to me. This is an unbelievably huge and daunting responsibility."

No One Is a Failure

Everything we feel and every disease is the result of a real trauma (that is experience), *never* of imagination as we may have been told. Therefore every response we have is real, with a real cause, and needs to be recognized.

Taking responsibility for how well you are in yourself begins with looking at what you are coping with. Who would start up a business without first considering all aspects and how viable they are? Or who would build a house without first finding out how to support the structure and keep the weather out? We have to consider just what we have experienced so far and what we are dealing with at present in all aspects of our lives. If we can see and feel what we are dealing with in our own life experience and the damage it has done to us we will not need to be disappointed in ourselves for not doing well enough.

What You Feel Is What You Are

It starts with acknowledgement, no hiding the facts and pretending it is better than it is, but the *truth as you feel it*. If you make a business plan that does not take into account certain factors it will never be achieved because you have left out some vital information. If you build a house without a proper foundation it will not be the house that you planned; it will change because you have not taken everything into account.

Consider any divorce case and you will have to acknowledge that the truth for one person can be different from the truth for another. Truth is not a fixed thing. Being true to yourself is *your* truth. What other people think you should be will not change how you really are, nor will what *you* think you should be. Whatever behavior you may choose to adopt, how you *feel* is how you *are*. You can pretend that you do not feel a certain way, or you can act as if you do not feel a certain way, but inside you will be feeling exactly what you are feeling. You can manipulate others but you cannot manipulate yourself.

THE EFFECTS OF REFLEXOLOGY

Reflexology treatment works to stimulate the body's systems so that they can function fully. When muscular tension is impeding the free functioning of a part of the body reflexology will work on that tension to enable it to release the contraction that has been held. When a muscle or muscles are not relaxing and contracting freely but are held in maintained contraction they will not be able to play their part fully in the metabolism of the muscles where energy is manufactured. Our muscles' activity produces energy, some of which is used in movement, more is used as heat to warm the body. Waste products from the muscular process are excreted through the venous system. If these waste products — which are toxins to the body — are not cleared fully the effect will be muscular stiffness and tension.

Physiologically certain specific effects can be seen as a result of reflexology treatment. Muscular tension will affect more than just the muscles. The supply of arterial (oxygenated) blood and venous blood (on its way back to the heart and lungs) and the nerve supply may all be constricted or reduced through long-term muscular tension. Treatment will allow the reflexes to enable the release of that tension, stimulating the muscles to let go and relax. It will also stimulate the release of the feelings held in the muscles that have been in a state of retained tension.

The circulation is improved so that waste products and toxins will be more effectively removed from the body via the venous blood and the lymphatic system. In the same way the supply of nutrients to all body parts will be enhanced by the increased flow of the blood supply. Increased activity of one organ may, and often will, have an effect leading to increased activity of other organs. For example, muscular activity results in better elimination of carbon dioxide and, in turn, the presence of this gas in the blood stimulates respiration. This results in a greater intake of oxygen, which stimulates the heart to beat more strongly and distribute the oxygenated blood to all the muscles (all tissues) where it is needed for the utilization of energy and elimination of waste.

How It Feels

The immediate results may be a feeling of relaxation, or alternately, of stimulation and increased energy and liveliness. People often go into a deep state of relaxation while receiving reflexology. This may make them feel very open, which lowers their defenses that help to protect them against the demands and attacks of the world. It is a good idea to be gentle with yourself after a treatment, preferably giving yourself time to assimilate the effects. It is certainly not wise to go straight into a noisy or demanding environment or situation. They will seem more stressful than usual while you are in an open and pliable state. It may also have the unfortunate effect of undoing the benefits of the treatment because you tense up to protect yourself.

Some people find that treatment stimulates a sluggish body into action — they feel a surge of energy and feel lively and energized throughout the day, or even the next few days.

BETTER OUT THAN IN

Sometimes, as toxins are eliminated from the body, people may experience some discomfort with their passing. This type of reaction will not last more than a few days and is the body's way of cleansing and healing itself, though this may not be what it feels like while it is happening. Today we are inclined to expect instant cures to any problem we experience rather than having patience as our body works out how to deal with the trouble. This is usually misguided. No illness comes without a cause, and the factors contributing to this cause build up over a period of time. Instant solutions rarely give the body time to deal with the cause and eliminate the problem. Rather they act as a band-aid, masking or covering up the visible signs of trouble. If you put a band-aid on top of a wound that has dirt in it the wound will fester and try to fight and clear away the dirt — it will not just heal up nicely. So, if you take medication that prevents a symptom from showing, the cause of that symptom will still, like the dirt in the cut, continue to fester away underneath — that is, *inside* your body.

HEALING REACTIONS

The elimination of troubles of the body is why people may experience what is known as a healing crisis, uncomfortable reactions when receiving reflexology, or any other alternative/complementary therapy. We call it a healing crisis because the body is going through a state of crisis in order to rid itself of what is making it less than well, and is acting to heal itself. A healing reaction will not last long, and afterward the person will invariably feel well — much better than before. This usually lasts: it is a healing, not just an alleviation of symptoms.

The type of response or reaction you may experience varies, but it will be a result of some pushing out of problems or toxins in the way that is appropriate for you and your individual body and life experience. It will be an elimination of some kind. For instance, a cold is your body's way of eliminating through the respiratory system; increased urination shows that the kidneys are working to cleanse your body; increased or loose bowel movements indicate elimination through the digestive system; a skin rash is a clearing out through the skin (which is an important and often overlooked organ of elimination that plays a key role in keeping the body healthy); a headache or dreams are the body/mind's way of throwing out things that are troubling it. A healing reaction is not a side effect — it is central to the body's process. Whatever the reaction, it will be passing; if it lasts more than a few days it will most likely be a condition that has become established for some reason rather than a reaction to treatment.

THE POOL

Imagine a pool that has become silted up when a stream has run low and the water flows slowly. Sediment of all kinds has collected at the bottom and around the edges. Stagnation has set in, with resulting growths. The process of decay moves in to clear up some of the dying matter. To stimulate cleansing and re-establish healthy growth and vitality spring floods are needed to flush quantities of clean water through the pool and clear away the debris that has restricted the life of the pool. This stirs up the silt at the bottom of the pool and the waters become muddy and chaotic for a while until the job is done and the water settles down again. Now that it is clear and bright you can see the pebbles at the bottom; plants flourish and fish dart about. Vibrant life has been restored. The process of a healing crisis is similar to this analogy.

GETTING IN TOUCH WITH YOUR FEELINGS

Reflexology treatment enables you to feel more clearly what you are already feeling. If you are a harassed single mother of three young children struggling to care for your family and to manage all the conflicting demands of your situation you may be very well aware of just what it is you are having to cope with. It is quite likely that reflexology treatment will make you feel blissfully relaxed and wiped out so that your overwhelming desire is to go home and put yourself to bed at the same time as your children and sleep.

If you have experienced severe emotional trouble that has caused you pain that you have never had an opportunity to talk about or to resolve, that you have dealt with by putting on a brave face, perhaps having held the family together and appeared cheerful for their sakes, you may find that treatment makes you more aware of the unresolved pain. You may feel "churned up" again as you realize the feelings that are still there. Treatment will give you an opportunity to feel how you are now and become more aware of what you *really* feel inside.

Every emotion has its physical manifestation. When we feel a strong emotion our bodies react in a certain way — particular muscles tense or relax accordingly, and in turn affect the functioning of the organs they work with. If you have tensed certain leg muscles while suffering from a shock it is quite possible, and even likely, that when you—maybe years later—become aware again of tension in those muscles you will subconsciously recall and relive the emotions you experienced at the time of the shock. This is called cellular memory. Memories recorded in our bodies in this way may date back to any time since conception. Of course, if they are precognitive (concerning events that happened before your powers of consciously recalling memories had developed in the brain, at around two and a half years) you may not be able to identify the cause, the actual happening, but you will be quite clear about the emotion you experienced at the time.

Psychosomatic

The effects of working the reflexes is psychosomatic. The word *psycho* is from the Greek *psyche*, meaning breath of life, the spirit or soul. Somatic is of the body, from the Greek word *soma*, meaning body. The two are interlinked like flame and fire. Each depends on and influences the other. So, the condition of the body affects the emotions just as physical diseases may have an emotional origin.

What Is Cure?

Treatment frees the body of impediment or restraint and enables the inner healing process to act fully. Impediment and restraint inhibit movement and restrict change, which is the natural state of life. When an illness is progressing and changes are taking place indicating movement, even if the condition seems to be worsening, as in a fever, the body is probably in control and waging an effective war on the invading forces. This, of course, depends on the individual specific circumstances and indications. It is when a condition becomes stuck and there is no change or progression that help is required. The body is indicating that it is not coping. Stagnation or lack of change is dangerous.

We have seen here how treatment acts on a physical and emotional level; it also acts on the subtle energy of the body. This is the energy flow around the body understood by meridian theory and central to the principles of acupuncture, homoeopathy, reflexology, shiatsu, and most complementary therapies. This is not the energy produced by muscular activity, but the subtle energy found in all matter. It helps explain the principle that the reflexes are linked in some way through the subtle energies to their corresponding organs, though not just or literally through a direct line through the nerves.

To sum up, treatment releases tension in the body and stimulates the various bodily systems. In the same way and at the same time, treatment affects emotional constrictions so that they may be released. Treatment also promotes the flow of the subtle energies around the body.

THE HOLISTIC APPROACH

Holistic comes from the Greek word *holos,* meaning whole, and holistic treatment takes into consideration the whole person. Reflexology approaches health, and each individual who comes for treatment, in a holistic way. The treatment focuses on the totality of the individual: their psychic and physical condition; their life situation and how they feel about things; their thoughts; how their mind works; and their particular experience of their condition.

Treatment is given to the whole person, not just for the specific condition that they are suffering from. Treatment is given for the whole body, not just for the part affected by the problem. In practice this means that rigid judgments are not to be made about the kind of treatment that should be given for the case. Treatment starts with a main focus and is adapted according to the patient's reactions. It also means that the practitioner keeps an open mind at all times and endeavors to listen fully to what the person has to say.

WORKING TO ESTABLISH BALANCE OR HOMEOSTASIS

The reflexologist's aim is to find a state of balance for the patient as a whole person—body, mind, and spirit. When one aspect is struggling, treatment aims to restore balance through renewed energy flow before the trouble spreads. If someone is dealing with problems that seem insurmountable they feel overwhelmed and fearful. They have negative thoughts that influence their bodies. This produces tensions, affecting the hormonal system, which is susceptible to mood changes. This in turn has an impression on the immune system. In this way the body's defense mechanism and circulation is constricted, as is the functioning of the whole body. Balance is lost between the systems and the flow of energy around the body, which somewhere, becomes congested and sluggish or uneasy. This imbalance creates favorable conditions for disease to move in, which results in further impaired functioning and discomfort or pain, which in turn gives rise to negative thoughts.

This cycle undermines the health of the whole organism and increasingly weakens the vital force, inhibiting the inner healing process. When congestion of emotions or body inhibits energy flow we feel increasingly cut off, separate in our trouble, as if the vital force of energy essential to life were being denied us. It is not possible to stop the flow of energy, but if we are out of balance and feel cut off then our body/mind/spirit will not be nurtured and maintained in health — which should be our natural state.

BODY, MIND AND SPIRIT — EACH INFLUENCING THE OTHER

When there is a problem in one part of the body the rest of the body is affected in some way—all parts being linked in the functioning of the whole. When an organ is malfunctioning it is not sufficient to isolate that part for treatment because it has a relationship with the surrounding and interconnected body parts, sometimes in ways we could not easily have predicted.

Similarly, when there is a physical illness the mental and emotional state of the person contribute to the cause and affect the progress of recovery. The state of the patient's feelings has a profound influence not just on the specific illness but on the whole body. This makes communication crucial in treatment. It is important to give patients a chance to say how they feel about their experience of the illness — what they feel is its cause and what they feel they most need to change in their lives. It is not unusual for people to remark to me while receiving reflexology treatment that this is the first time anyone has listened to them and the first time they have been asked what *they* feel is the cause of their condition.

TALKING ABOUT YOURSELF

If you visit a professional reflexology practitioner you will be asked some questions about your lifestyle and medical background that enables the practitioner to decide on the best treatment for you. This is also to protect you from the wrong treatment based on lack of knowledge about your particular state of health. For example, if you have diabetes the treatment must be given with great care—not right after a meal—and with the knowledge and monitoring of your doctor. During treatment how much you talk is up to you. Some people use the time to air their problems, to pour out what is troubling them; others go into a deep state of relaxation and do not wish to talk much; yet others enjoy a bit of both, but do not want to go into depth about how they feel.

HOW LONG AND HOW OFTEN?

Your practitioner should speak to you about his suggestions for a course of treatment based on the information you have given him and his findings during your session. He should also give you some idea of how long is needed to bring about the changes you desire. This should be reviewed in the light of any progress and any new decisions should be made together at each session.

CHOOSING YOUR REFLEXOLOGIST

The best way to find a reflexology practitioner is by word of mouth. However, you have to take into account whether your criteria would be the same as those of the person making the recommendation. Of course, this does not tell you anything about the standard of training the practitioner has achieved.

SELF-HELP

If you are planning to learn and use reflexology for self-help, or within your family and circle of friends without professional training, it is essential that you read the following chapter. You will then be aware of what is involved and be responsible in recognizing when you need to know more, and when it is safe to use basic techniques.

WHAT ARE YOU AIMING FOR AND INTENDING TO DO?

Reflexology is a therapy that is well suited to self-help. It is also something that you can learn to do relatively easily so that you can work the feet of your family and friends.

The techniques of foot massage and pressure point therapy can be acquired by anyone willing to learn with care, sensitivity, and awareness. All you have to do is develop a "feel" for doing it. You need to work with these qualities and make one golden rule for yourself: *the only thing that matters is to learn what the feet are telling you, and to follow their lead.* Let the state of the feet and their response dictate to you how you work. In this way you can offer yourself and your family valuable relief when tired or stressed; perform a deeply relaxing experience; and help in maintaining good health and preventing illness.

Focus On Your Partner

It is essential to follow what the feet are showing you and to listen to the person without making personal judgments about what she may be telling you, and without giving advice. Whether you are a professional or not, your job as a reflexologist is to work the feet, to respond to what they indicate, and to consider the entirety of your partner.

You then are playing an active part in working the feet and a passive (supporting) role by listening to and acknowledging what your partner says. This is important whether you think she is "right" or not, or believe she could do better if only she could see it. A reflexology session, whether given by a professional or done informally at home among friends, is *never* an opportunity to enjoy voicing your own knowledge and perceptions. Rather it is a creative interchange during which you use your hands to massage and release tensions, your ears to listen, and your heart to care from a position of genuine respect for your partner. (Not from a feeling of doing good or of any superiority).

For the person receiving it is a chance to relax and be nurtured — a time for themselves, to speak or remain quiet as they wish. Because reflexology touches not only physical but emotional tensions (felt in the body through muscular tensing as well as in the mind) it is important to keep the session centered on the person receiving. This is an invaluable guide. If your partner chooses to talk about something you can follow because the subject is appropriate — *they* have brought it up. Again, it is not appropriate for you to raise a subject. Keep your own interests to yourself until afterward when you meet on equal terms and you are no longer in a care-giving position.

Professional Treatment or at Home?

The difference between receiving reflexology at home from a friend and going to a professional reflexologist is obviously the latter's background knowledge about how reflexology works; how the body is structured and works (anatomy and physiology); and what can go wrong (pathology). A professional knows the causes of various conditions, and how the various bodily systems can react to problems (integrated biology). She is expert at working the reflexes and energy pathways for particular conditions (the practice of reflexology).

The Professional's Expertise and Judgment

The practitioner's knowledge and experience will be necessary when somebody has an established or long-term (chronic) condition or when the patient is in a fragile and therefore precarious state of health. Treatment should be carried out in conjunction with any other professionals involved. Generally, the longer a disease or condition has been present the more treatment will be needed to bring about permanent change. Reflexology treatment is cumulative, and the practitioner will have to use his professional judgment in order to decide how frequently sessions are needed, how long a course of treatment should last, and what the prognosis is for improvement. The practitioner will explain this to the client and will review it and discuss progress at regular intervals. To achieve major changes in health and well-being this expertise is crucial.

Reflexology at Home — Doing It Yourself

Reflexology performed at home can be wonderfully beneficial in encouraging and maintaining a state of well-being. It is very relaxing. It stimulates the body to function more fully and it can provide some relief for someone under a lot of pressure or who is suffering an everyday ailment.

Amazing results can be achieved by anyone who is aware and sensitive enough to respond to what is found on the feet. In one respect, all that is necessary is to take into account what the feet are indicating—whether you know what the reflex is or not. If you work in this manner, keep your wits about you, and remain sensitive to your partner you can achieve a lot. You won't cause any harm if you *always* follow the lead of the person you are working with. This means that if she shows or says that it feels uncomfortable or painful you should immediately respond by working more lightly and gently around that place. If possible still work it as for long as necessary.

LISTENING TO YOUR PARTNER

If your partner has a headache and you find tender spots around the neck of the toes and in the instep, work those carefully and try to release some of the tension there rather than working on the head of the toes because you know he has a *head*ache. The head may not be the problem — it may just be the outlet for the pain. This applies to any condition: The main area of trouble may not lie on the site of the named symptom.

"Trouble" may be tenderness or discomfort felt by the recipient, or tightness, deposits, lumps, or strands of congestion felt by the person giving the massage. It may also be visual signs indicating imbalance — for example, hard skin, corns, callouses, verrucas.

PROTECTING YOU BOTH FROM INFECTION

Wherever there is broken skin or infection the area should always be covered to protect both of you so that cross-infection does not occur.

WHAT YOU NEED TO GIVE A REFLEXOLOGY TREATMENT

Before giving a treatment always ask whether your partner has any illness or is going to the doctor for any disorder. You must protect anyone you work with, and yourself, from the distress or even danger of exacerbating any problem they may have. This is actually unlikely to happen, but in cases where it *could*, it is *absolutely crucial*. Without training you will not know what these problems are. Therefore, make it a golden rule to always check with your partner before you start.

Take the example of someone with diabetes. If you gave a reflexology treatment to a diabetic without knowledge of his condition and its implications you might well give the treatment after lunch or in the evening after a meal. You would not know that treatment should not be given to diabetics after eating because the balance of the blood sugar level is very precarious. If you inadvertently stimulated the pancreas the levels of insulin could become dangerous and a severe reaction could result.

What to Do If Your Partner Has a Medical Condition

If your partner is under a doctor's care for any reason you should only give a light foot massage. If she wishes to receive reflexology she should consult a professional reflexologist. The reflexologist will not perform any reflexology until the patient has informed her doctor. In this way, the doctor has a chance to pass on any information she feels the reflexologist should know.

Remember that wherever there is broken skin or an infection the area should be covered to protect both of you from cross-infection.

Position Your Partner Comfortably

Make sure that the room you are using is warm and quiet. The position for treatment should be a comfortable one, usually reclining, and in such a way that you can see each other's faces and talk without effort. Your partner's back must be comfortable and well supported, not folded up or kinked. This is very important because energy must be able to flow freely up and down the spine. The head should have a pillow or soft cushion under it, and most particularly, the neck must be supported as part of the spine and not under any strain. Place a pillow under your partner's knees so that they are bent. This will facilitate the flow of the blood supply to the legs and feet and not put any strain on the legs.

You may use a sofa, propping your partner up diagonally across it so that you can reach his feet at one corner, positioning them as above. You may be able to find something to support the legs adequately if the person sits in an armchair. An alternative position that you can use anywhere is to have your partner lying on the floor on something comfortable. Support the head on a pillow with his legs elevated and resting on a soft surface of a stool or chair, his neck and legs supported as described above.

Position Yourself Comfortably

You yourself must be comfortable if you are going to effectively work without getting tired and strained. To do this you must be seated at the correct height so that you can reach the feet with your hands and see what you are doing without straining your back. A pile of cushions or a low stool on the floor is probably the best seat for you. As long as you are comfortable and you can reach your partner and see, any variation will do.

Keeping Warm

You will need to have a blanket on hand so that if your partner becomes chilly, which often happens as she relaxes and her temperature drops, you can cover her. Have a warm soft towel to cover the foot you are not working on to keep it warm.

Materials

Your partner's feet should be clean and dry. You do not need any materials. However, if you find the feet you are working on become moist or sweaty it is useful to shake powder sparingly on to your hands before touching the feet again. This helps you to massage without sticking to the skin. Oil is not used in reflexology because it is slippery and makes it difficult to put pressure on a precise reflex point. Talc-free baby powder or arrowroot are good. If you use talcum powder, use it sparingly. Reflexologists generally avoid it because it has been shown to be mildly carcinogenic. If you need to wipe over the feet use a cotton wool dipped in a little diluted calendula lotion. Calendula is a homeopathic tincture made from the marigold plant and is gentle but antiseptic. It can be bought at health stores supplying homeopathic preparations.

When all the reflexes have been worked it feels soothing and most enjoyable to end your treatment with oils that facilitate smooth and flowing massage as well as moisten and nourish the feet. Any base vegetable oil is suitable—almond oil is particularly good. If you have and use essential oils, add a few drops to the base oil. This should be done with extreme caution, however, and not unless your partner is also familiar with essential oils — they can be damaging or dangerous if used without knowledge of their properties.

A Pleasurable Experience

A reflexology treatment is a wonderfully relaxing and pleasurable experience. To make sure that it will be both of these things it is important that you are both comfortable and that the room is warm and free of interruptions (telephone ringing, people walking in and out, children or pets disrupting). People are often embarrassed about the state of their feet. They should be reassured that anyone who does reflexology meets feet of all shapes, sizes, and conditions. Feet with problems do not come as a surprise.

FOOT MASSAGE

Having your feet massaged is a soothing and very personal experience that is wonderfully relaxing and leaves you feeling peaceful, calm and nurtured. Stimulating the reflexes, which we will come to in the next chapter, is given within this framework. It is essential that you massage the feet well in order to relax and prepare them, to get your partner used to your touch, and to gain her trust and confidence.

Always wash your hands before you start to work and immediately as you finish so that you do not spread any infection. Also, it is good to prepare yourself mentally to give and, at the end, to recognize that you have completed this particular act of giving. Washing your hands symbolically focuses your attention on this. It is useful to clear your mind beforehand of your own concerns and afterward to clear your mind of any intimate feelings you may have picked up from your partner, to recognize that the special contact you have had is now over and you are back on an everyday equal footing.

You may prefer to sit quietly for a moment by your partner before you make contact and begin to massage. But make sure that you clear your mind before you start and when you finish. Take care that your hands are warm because it is not at all pleasant to be suddenly touched on the exposed skin of your feet, which are usually covered, by a pair of cold hands.

Massage Techniques

Massage techniques are usually referred to in French terms. The French term *effleurage* is known in reflexology as stroking movements, which is exactly what they are. Although the term stroking movements describes the action, *effleurage* is a pleasant sounding word to use.

It is not easy to teach very specific movements using the written word, with only pictures to illustrate them. What is more important than learning a variety of prescribed movements is to get a feel for a group of movements that you can use and adapt.

When you are ready to begin let your hands come down gently and slowly onto your partner's feet and rest them there for a short time so that you can feel the temperature, texture, and tone, and to "tune in" to the person. This allows him time to adjust to you. Then gently start to move your hands in flowing movements down or around the feet. There is not a great deal you can do on both feet at once, but it is good to do this for a short time to make an introduction.

When you are working one foot at a time use one hand to support the foot you are working on and the other to perform the movements. You may support the foot between your two hands as they both work together. Either way, it is very important that the foot being massaged is fully supported in a reassuring and comfortable hold, neither flopping about nor being held too tightly or pulled. So the first thing for you to pay attention to, before figuring out the massage movements, is how you are going to use your holding hand.

Massage movements fall into categories or types. I think of them as families. There are those that aim to soothe and relax; others that work to relax specific parts; and others whose purpose is to stimulate the tissues of the feet and encourage circulation.

1) STROKING OR EFFLEURAGE

For relaxation, stroking movements are used extensively — they are flowing and soothing. There are a number of ways in which you can use this type of movement.

a) Run your hands one after another down the top of the foot from the top of the ankle to the end of the toes.

b) Run your fingertips around and around the ankle bones smoothing the skin and tissues as you go.

c) Run your fingers down the sides of the foot from ankle to toes, one hand on each side — this feels a bit like water flowing down the foot.

d) Holding the foot you are working on with the hand that is on the big toe side, gently but securely use the palm and fingers of the other hand to massage around and around over the broad flat surface on the top of the foot lying between the little toes and the ankle.

e) Any variation you can make up that has a basic stroking movement is good to try out.

These techniques are not laid down in stone, but rather have evolved based on the principles outlined above. They can always be developed further. It is good to follow your hands and try out your own movements.

2) SPREADING MOVEMENTS

Also relaxing, but aiming to warm the tissues and stimulate the circulation as well, are spreading movements. With your fingers, and especially fingertips, you smooth and feel through the tissues to relax both the surface and the muscles. These movements should be done slowly with feeling.

a) Hold the sides of one foot with your hands so that your thumbs rest side by side on top of the foot pointing toward the leg, tips on the top of the ankle. Gripping firmly, but not hard, with your palms on the sides of the foot, gradually draw the thumbs sideway from the center of the foot toward the edges. Repeat this several times, each time starting a little farther down the foot toward the toes. In this way you will cover the top of the foot. Aim to have the entire length of the thumbs in contact with the top of the foot. Repeat the procedure once or twice.

b) Starting in exactly the same position, this time let the thumbs remain still, holding the foot on top while you draw the fingers across the sole of the foot, sideway to the edge, moving them all together. Repeat this several times, each time starting a little farther down the foot toward the toes. Continue until you reach the base of the toes. You are working from the heel down toward the toes. Repeat as above.

c) Next, reverse the position of your hands so that your thumbs are on the sole and your fingers meet across the top of the foot. While you hold the ball of the foot massage deeply with your thumbs across the whole of this area under all five toes.

d) Massage up the backs of the toes with your thumbs, running your thumbs up from the base of the toes to the tops. Do this while holding the ball of the foot with your hands on each side of the foot. Run your thumbs up the back of

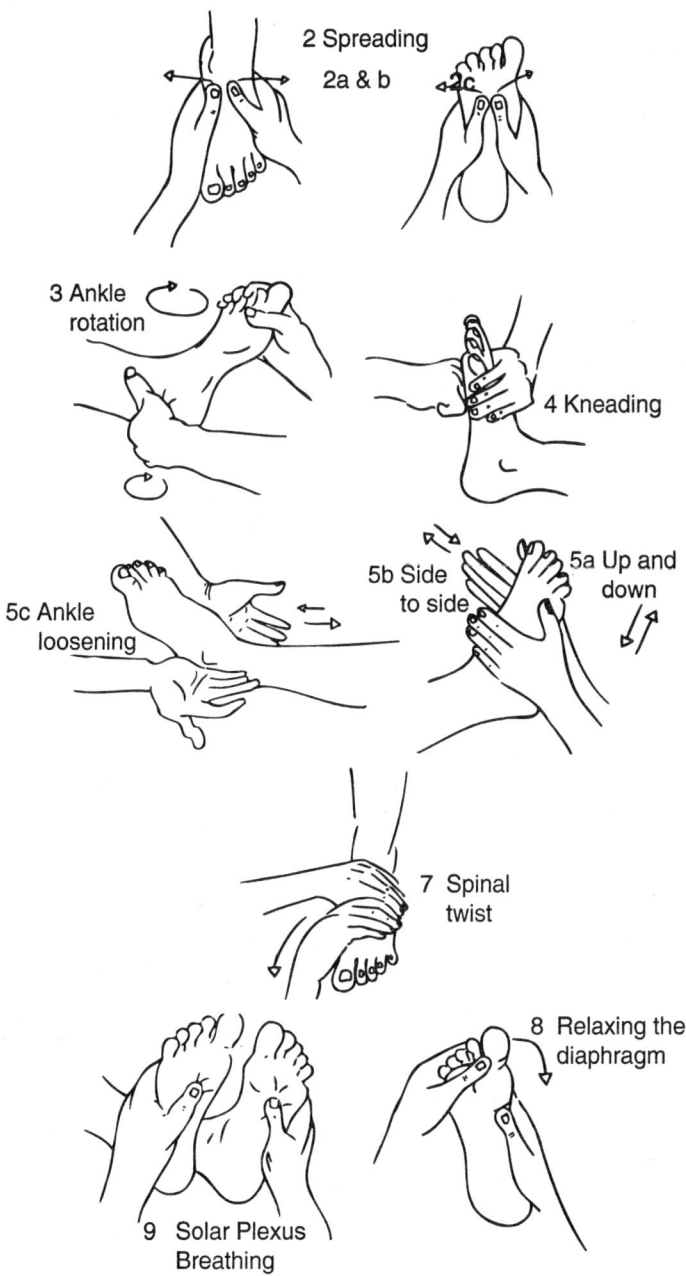

Illustration 3
Some Massage Movements

each toe one thumb after another; do this several times on each toe.

3) ANKLES

Ankle Rotation   Ankle rotation should be done early on to open up the blood supply to the foot and relax the entire ankle, which could be called the gateway to the foot. The blood supply to and from the foot and the nerves all have to pass through this area. If the muscles are tight, as they often are, then essential supplies will be restricted. This movement will help to relax the entire pelvic area: the base of the spine, the lower back muscles, the hip joints, and the pelvic floor.

Cup the heel in the palm of your supporting hand and hold the ball of the foot with your other hand. Using the hand that is on the outer side of the foot place it on the ball of the foot under the little toes — fingers on the top surface of the foot, thumb on the ball on the sole. Rotate the foot clockwise for several turns, exercising it enough to challenge it, but *never* forcing the foot. *Feel* your way through the circles. Both hands move — the upper hand leads while the lower hand joins in subtly, following the leading hand so that you can hardly see it move. Your hands move rather like the hands of a clock: the upper hand being the minute hand and moving more than the lower hand, which is the hour hand that moves ever so slightly. Do this for several turns and then repeat, turning counterclockwise.

Ankle Stretch   Hold the foot in the same way as you did in the ankle rotation. Stretch the foot downward so that the toe is pointed as far as it will comfortably go. Next, push the foot back toward the leg so that the toes point upward as far as they will comfortably go. Repeat if you wish.

4) KNEADING

Knead the sole, holding one foot at a time securely with one hand. With the other hand made into a fist, massage with the front of the fist (the lower portion of your fingers, not with the knuckles), working the entire sole just as if you were kneading bread. This should be a deep, slow, rhythmical movement. This stroke is particularly useful when working the heel on the sole where it is hard and padded — here you may use the knuckles of the second joint of the fingers to relax deep into the heel where both the sciatic and the pelvic reflexes lie.

5) STIMULATING MOVEMENTS

To stimulate the circulation, loosen tension in the muscles, and soften the tissues, vigorous, fast movements are used. For these, both hands work together, one on either side of the foot.

Up and Down and Side to Side   Cradling the foot between your hands, move your hands vigorously *up and down* the sides of the foot from heel to toes and back. In the same position, now roll the foot between your hands so that it rolls from *side to side.*

Ankle Loosening   After doing the above, work up behind the ankle bone with the sides of your hands, palms facing upward, stimulating and relaxing the sides of the heel. This is also quite a fast movement. Do not bump the ankle bone.

6) ROTATE ALL THE TOES

Using your working hand to hold the toes firmly without pinching them, rotate all the toes, holding the foot securely with the standard hold on the ball of the foot. This loosens the toes and increases flexibility while relaxing the neck muscles.

7) THE SPINAL TWIST

The spinal twist is used to relax the important spinal reflex that runs down the foot on the instep. Sitting to one side of your partner's feet, facing across them, place your hands side by side resting on the top of the ankle, fingers on top with index fingers touching, and thumbs underneath on the sole. Hold the top hand (on the ankle) *still*, while slowly and rhythmically running the other hand to and fro across the top of the foot and around the instep, as if you were ironing — using the flat of your hand and fingers. (When you reach the instep run your hand firmly and surely around it and back again the other way.) Your working hand keeps moving, sliding to and fro across the top of the foot, while the holding hand remains still, supporting it.

Next, move both hands forward a little and repeat the action. In this way travel a little farther downward toward the toes with each horizontal line (keeping the hands together, but not moving both hands at the same time) so that after a while your hand will reach the base of the toes. (Remember when if you iron without any pressure you do not iron out the creases.) You need sufficient pressure to iron out any tensions held in the muscles, but do it without dragging the skin. If you find the skin is dragging under your hand slow down a little and allow it time to slide out naturally from underneath. You may need to use a little powder to facilitate easy movement if the foot becomes moist and warm.

8) The Diaphragm

The diaphragm should be worked to ease tension. It runs along the base of the ball of the foot where there is a change of color and texture, between the ball (which takes our weight in contact with the ground) and the instep, which is not padded in the same way. You can work this with your thumb in two possible ways.

a) Holding the foot with the standard hold, position your working hand so that the thumb rests on the base of the ball where the instep begins (sole) and your fingers lie on top of the foot. Now, with your holding hand bring the foot down to press onto your thumb and lift it off again.

Move the thumb a step sideway and repeat. This movement is rather like pulling tap beer with a proper big handle down and up again. In this way work right along the diaphragm.

b) You may also relax the diaphragm by holding the foot in the same hold and working into the diaphragm by rotating your working thumb firmly but sensitively, one spot at a time, along the diaphragm line (fingers on top of the foot).

9) The Solar Plexus

The solar plexus lies on the diaphragm line. You can locate it by placing your hand on top of the foot and squeezing gently so that the pad crumples up — the solar plexus reflex lies in the dip at the center of this. The solar plexus is a sort of spaghetti junction of nerves supplying the abdomen and is referred to as the nerve switchboard, or sometimes as the abdominal brain. It is the primary center for collecting stress and nervousness.

Place one hand on each foot (right hand on right foot and left on left), with the ball of your thumbs resting on the solar plexus reflex and your hands around the outside of each foot, with the fingertips resting behind on the top of the foot.

Ask your partner to breathe in, and as they do, gently press in with your thumbs. As they breathe out, simultaneously release the pressure of your thumbs.

Repeat several times.

Using the Massage Techniques

It is not possible without practical demonstration to give a clear description of precise massage techniques. Neither is it necessary. Massage was used long before people invented and named techniques. It is used today all over the world spontaneously and instinctively when we touch a hurt part of our bodies or caress a baby or small child or show physical affection. A massage in Thailand today will be at once similar and different to one received in this country or to one given in Bali. And of course two massages received in this country will vary as much as the practitioners themselves.

Use the written directions and illustrations in this book as you feel appropriate, with awareness of the person who is receiving the massage. The ideas are intended to start you off and to show you some of the differing types of massage movements. The best and most enjoyable thing you can do next is to build on this basic information and improvise, following your hands and intuition, trying different movements out. *Above all, get a feel for giving massage and always give it with awareness of the person to whom you are giving.*

REFLEXOLOGY TECHNIQUES AND LEARNING TO GIVE A TREATMENT

Once you have thoroughly prepared your partner's feet with a good massage you will be ready to work the reflex points. The basic reflexology technique is thumb walking. This is used to cover all the reflexes, working the whole of the feet. Remember that reflexology is not only holistic because it takes into account the whole person, but also because the practitioner works directly on the whole person by working the whole of the feet.

THE TECHNIQUES

To start with, you decide which hand is going to be the supporting hand (or holding hand) and which is the working hand. Generally you will work most effectively with the hand that is nearest to the reflex you are covering. The other hand will be your supporting hand. Some people are so strongly right- or left-handed, though, that they adapt this. It is good to try to use your hands as equally as possible. This enables you to access the reflexes efficiently. Try it with an open mind, accepting that it will feel fairly strange until you accustom yourself and your fingers to the work. You may as well endeavor to learn proper practices from the start.

The Supporting Hand

The job of the supporting hand is to give security to the person you are working with. It must convey surety and reassurance: that they are "in good hands." This hand also has a very important part to play in holding the foot still to enable you to work and reach the reflexes. It is not at all relaxing, and indeed is very uncomfortable to have your foot yanked around as if it were not attached to a feeling human being. Therefore, the two hands work together to ensure your partner's comfort while facilitating your access to the points on the feet.

Thumb Walking

It is important to master the technique of thumb walking because this is the key to giving effective treatments. It is also sometimes called caterpillar walking and you will see why if you look at Illustration 5.

If you have ever played the children's rhyme "Two fat gentlemen met in a lane, bowed most politely, bowed once again. How do you do? How do you do? How do you do again?" you will know how to do the basic thumb walking movement. It is just the same as the finger play for this rhyme, where you hold both hands up in front of you, palms facing you and thumbs on the outside, fingers curled loosely into a fist.

With each "How do you do," one thumb bends at the first joint, as if it were a fat gentleman bowing. Practice it in this position, alternate thumbs or together. Aim to keep your arm and the rest of your hand relaxed: all the action is in the thumb and it is important that you do not tense up the muscles of your hand or you will become very stiff and tired. You will also be less sensitive to feeling the response in your partner's reflexes. This is very important because a great deal of sensitivity is required to do a good job, to not overstimulate or temporarily damage any of the sensitive reflexes you will be working on.

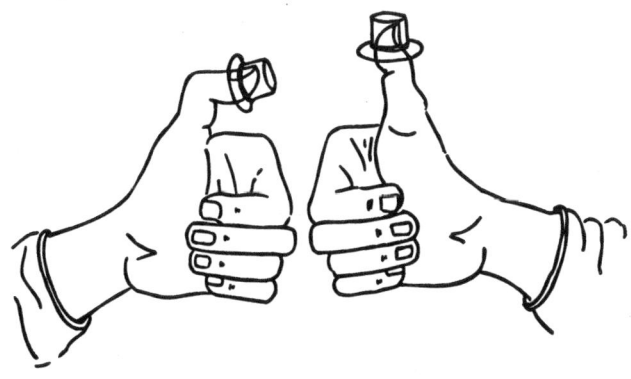

Illustration 4
How to Use Your Thumbs "Two Fat Gentlemen"

When you feel you have roughly grasped this technique try to apply it to your own hand. Have one hand in front of you, palm facing you. Rest the thumb of your other (working) hand on the padded part at the bottom of the palm (of the first hand) on a line with your little finger (just above the wrist). Place the fingers of your working hand behind the first hand for support and anchorage. Now press down with your thumb tip and then stretch it out so that your thumb slides forward a fraction and the pad of the thumb lands on the place where the tip was pressing before. Look at Illustration 5 again. Repeat this step. When you can do this consecutively you are thumb walking.

FINGER WALKING

Later on you will need to try the above with a finger — the index or middle — as sometimes it will be easier to access points with a finger than a thumb. This is finger walking. (Thumb walking is the main technique used, however.)

There are two other important reflexology techniques: rotating and pin-pointing.

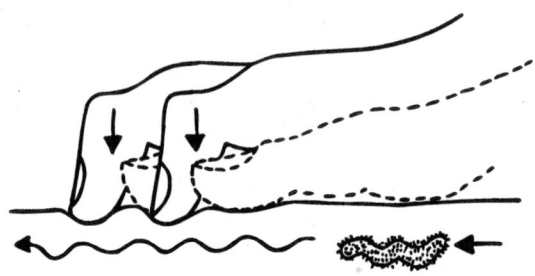

Illustration 5
Thumbs Walking — Like a Caterpillar

ROTATING

Rotating is exactly as it sounds: positioning your thumb or finger on the reflex you are about to work, rotate it gently on the spot, feeling carefully as you do so, and being careful not to press so hard that it causes pain. *This is very important — you have to find out what is acceptable for each person.* For some people a very light touch may be uncomfortable, whereas for others you may use quite a lot of pressure. Also, it is important for you to know that some reflexes on a person's foot may be excruciatingly tender whereas other points will be much less so.

PIN-POINTING

Pin-pointing is a specialist technique for working certain deep reflexes that cannot be successfully accessed any other way. Try this out on your hand as you did the thumb walking. Position your hands as before: have one hand in front of you, palm facing you. Rest the thumb of your other (working) hand on the padded part at the bottom of the palm below your little finger (just above the wrist). This time tilt your working thumb onto the inner corner (the corner next to the finger) and let the top thumb joint be bent — see Illustration 6.

Now feel into the fleshy pad of the hand you are working on, using quite a lot of pressure. If you were doing this on a specific reflex point you would be checking for any response and ascertaining whether there was any discomfort. The second part of the movement is to pull down deeply into the tis-

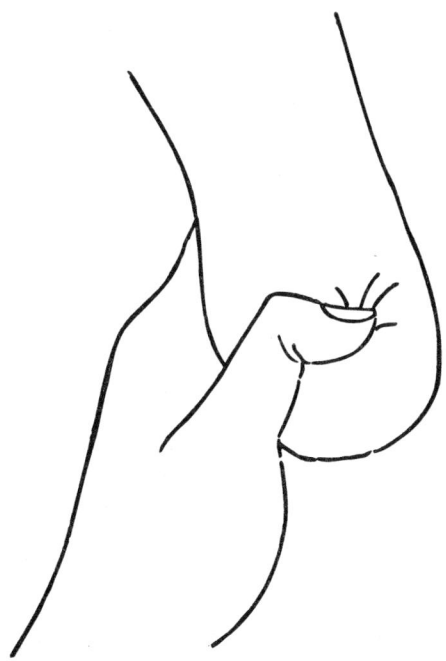

Illustration 6
The Position for Pin-Pointing

sues underneath the surface with a short, distinct movement, and then release it. The classic way to describe this movement is the "hook in and back up" technique, which is just as it sounds. The "backward" movement refers to moving deeply down into the tissues below your thumb. Quite often when working the appropriate reflexes in this way you will find that someone who has experienced little or no sensation during the first part of the technique will have a very definite response to the deep movement of the pin-pointing.

As with thumb walking and rotating, it is essential that you check your partner's response before applying firm pressure. Remember that some people will be very sensitive while others may take quite a lot of pressure. Also bear in mind that the same person's sensitivity may well vary from one time to the next. Pin-pointing is only used on thickly padded parts such as the heel.

Holding

In the previous chapter we looked at movements for giving massage and in this chapter we have learned specific reflexology techniques. There is one other way of using your hands that may simply be called holding, but which is very important. How often when you have hurt yourself, or when you have a pain, have you placed your hands on the sore place for comfort and it has felt a little better? Most people do this instinctively and do not think about why they are doing it. When a child, or an adult, is upset, have you held them, for comfort, until they feel a little better?

It doesn't matter why it works as long as it does, but what is actually happening is a transfer of energy. So when someone or a body part has received a shock or trauma (be it physical or emotional) the person will feel depleted, wounded. The healing contained in a good touch conveys warmth and comfort through transferring energy to the wounded part, thus enabling it to begin to regenerate or heal.

Using the Techniques to Stimulate Healing within the Body

When you thumb walk or rotate on the reflexes of the feet you stimulate the energy that flows around the body, repairing and healing wherever there is damage or lack of full functioning. When parts are not functioning at their optimum level, or when there is a specific problem, we call this imbalance. When you hold a part of the foot that seems to be particularly sensitive or painful, or which you feel drawn to hold, you are helping the energy that flows through all of us to flow to the part that particularly needs to repair and heal.

Practice this way of using your hands as well as the more active movements if it feels good to you because it is very valuable.

Energy Flow Along the Spine

When you work the spinal reflex, place your hands or fingertips at either end of the reflex and hold for as long as feels right. You may position your hands beside the big toe nail on the outside of the toe, on the spinal line, and on the inside of the ankle between the ankle bone and the heel (the coccyx). In this way you will enable the flow of energy along the spine (through the reflexes) between the chakras from the crown to the base. Or, you may place your hands, one on the neck of the big toe on the outside and the other, as before, on the inside of the ankle on the coccyx reflex, to stimulate the energy flow along the spine and central nervous system in the spinal cord. Reflexologists often call this linking.

Putting Theory into Practice

When you have mastered the reflexology techniques and feel comfortable giving a foot massage you will be ready to put the two together. Prepare and position yourself and your partner as described in Chapter 10. Then begin by giving a good foot massage. Next thumb walk up each of the five zones on each foot, one foot at a time, from the heel to the toes. This is a good way to begin because it is straightforward, although it will be necessary to lift the foot you are working on with your holding hand under the heel in order to reach the lower portion of the foot at the start of each zone.

Then go on to working the whole of the feet, following the routine (Illustration 10). It is always important to work all the reflexes, not just to work those that seem to relate to any problem or condition your partner may have. Neither practitioners nor doctors are always aware of the underlying causes or contributing factors behind someone's condition. *If you highlight or work only the reflexes relating to the trouble you may not find or aid the reflexes that will enable the body to fully heal itself.*

For example, you can actually cause a headache to become much worse by working the head area, thereby stimulating the part that is already congested and carrying a lot of pressure.

What is needed in this situation is to draw or drain away the congested energy and fullness from the troubled head down through the body to relieve the tension and pressure. If you draw energy that has collected in the head, which is causing the pressure, down through the body allowing it to become a balanced part of the energy flow around the body, or draw it down to the feet where it may pass harmlessly into the ground, you will help the body move through to recovery.

In Chapter 14 we will go right through a full reflexology treatment with Illustrations 11 and 12 at the end of the book to refer to. Here we are still building up a method of working and experimenting to get a feel for reflexology.

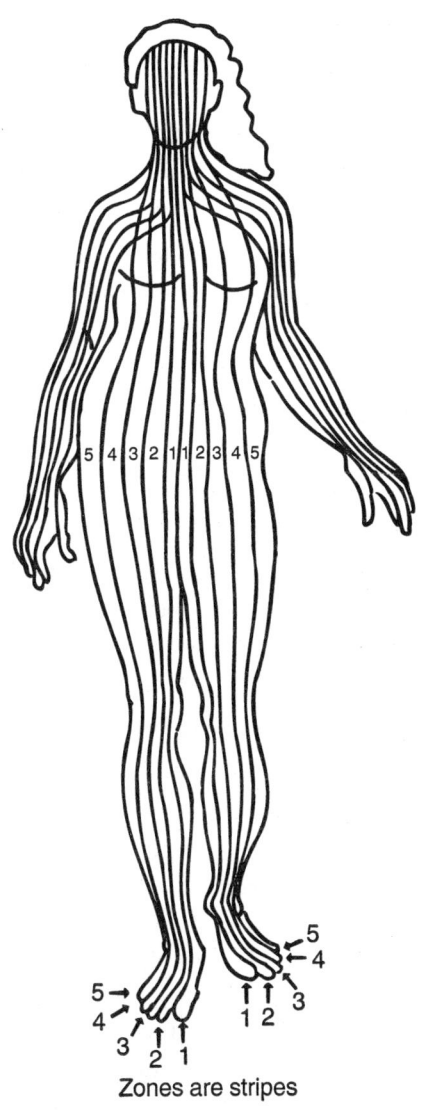

Illustration 7
The Zones

The Zones

When William Fitzgerald and others rediscovered the effects of sedating or stimulating one part of the body to influence another area they believed that the parts that related to one another lay along one of five zones. Any body part lying in zone five can be affected by another in that zone. The relationships are distinct to the zones, which each run symmetrically and uniformly throughout the whole body — see Illustration 7.

It seems very clear that relationships between parts affecting each other do indeed lie along pathways running vertically through our body, and that these pathways are symmetrical. Understanding the meridians shows that these pathways follow the general line of the zones, but are rather more complex, bending and zig-zaging within the general outline of the zones. See Illustration 8.

Zone theory theorizes that relationships exist within the body along specific lines. Meridian theory details what these relationships are and how various organs may relate to each other across the body's systems. This theory offers a wealth of information as to how the body works and how problems may develop.

Transverse Zones

There are also transverse zones that divide the body into areas — see Illustration 9. These zones are between the shoulderline (running under the toes), the diaphragm (separating the ball of the foot from the instep), the waistline, and the heel line. To identify the waistline, run your fingers down the outside of the foot until you feel and see the protruding end of the fifth metatarsal bone — about halfway down. Take this prominence as your marker for the waistline, making an imaginary line right across the foot to the instep — this line is the waist. Apart from the waistline,

DISCOVER REFLEXOLOGY   77

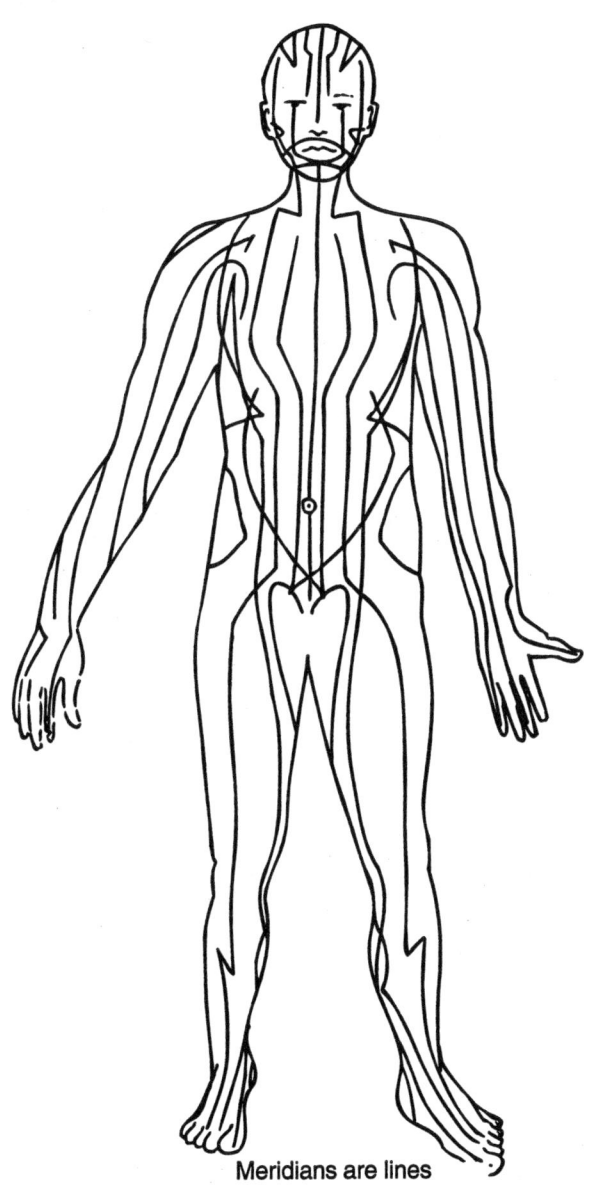

Illustration 8
The Meridians

these lines are usually easy to see from the changes in texture and color of the foot. The ball and heel are padded and usually have more color than the instep, which is pale.

THE REFLEX AREAS

When you give a reflexology treatment you will be concentrating on areas of the body one at a time. Look again at Illustration 9.

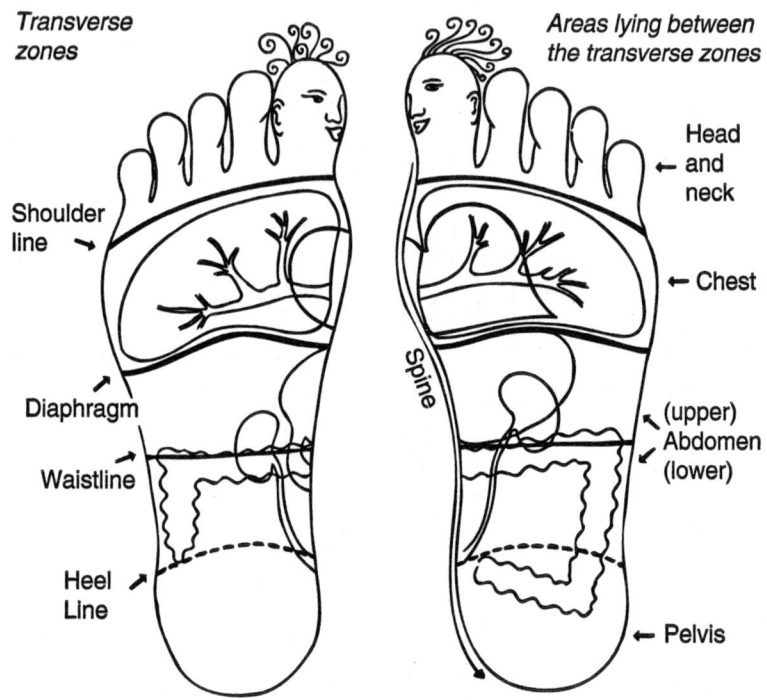

Illustration 9
The Transverse Zones

THE HEAD AND NECK

First work the toes thoroughly, stimulating the reflexes to the head and neck. Have a look at Illustration 9 and see where these lie. In addition, the toes have the beginnings or the ends of five of the six major meridians that lie in the feet. It is good to work the toes thoroughly to relieve the many congestions that tend to collect around these meridian ends, and to release the many congestions that are held in the neck, particularly, and the head.

The Chest

Next concentrate on the chest area, which lies on the top and sole of the ball of the foot — see Illustrations 11 and 12 for the specific reflexes.

The Abdomen

The abdomen contains many complex vital organs that are the processing plant of our body: digesting or converting the food and liquids we eat and drink into the substances from which we are made. Look at Illustrations 11 and 12 again.

We are familiar with most of the visceral organs, even if we do not fully understand their functioning, but the ileo-caecal valve deserves a mention here. It features, often prominently, in reflexology. This reflex is often painful or congested when worked. The ileo-caecal valve can be found in many chronic conditions. It is the opening (a one-way valve) between the small and large intestines and can often become a bit of a bottleneck, which leads to congestion.

The Pelvis

This is represented on the heel, both on the sole and on the sides of the heel, and on top of the ankle and around it. See Illustrations 11 and 12.

The Spine

The spine runs along the instep and curves up along the bony edge underneath the ankle bone, as shown in Illustrations 11 and 12.

All of these represent the right side of the body on the right foot and the left side of the body on the left foot.

The Sequence of Treatment

When you work, greet your partner and her feet with massage to relax and prepare them. Then concentrate first on the reflex areas on the right foot (see Illustration 10) while the left foot is warmly wrapped in a soft towel. Use massage throughout, between working the reflexes. When you have completed the right foot, wrap it up snugly in the towel and start to massage and work the reflex areas of the left foot, again using massage in between. Finish by giving a good massage to both feet to relax the body after any discomfort that may have been felt in the reflexes. This gives a sense of well-being to your partner.

Some reflexologists work from one area to the next across the body, covering the toes first on the left and then on the right and so on for the chest area, abdominal, pelvic, and spinal areas. I find this disturbing, as do my patients, because you have to keep uncovering one foot and then the other. Certainly the chest lies across both feet, but the organs of the abdomen are not symmetrical and differ from right to left. On the other hand, the meridians run vertically down the feet. Classically, reflexologists work one foot at a time.

Work the right foot first and then the left. The right side of the body is controlled by the left side of the brain, which is the analytical part of the brain that deals with abstract and external ideas. The left side of the body is controlled by the right side of the brain, which is the more artistic and intuitive part and deals more with inner feelings.

Experience shows that people often want to chat during the treatment of the first foot, and that they commonly go into a deep state of relaxation while the left foot is being worked on, becoming quiet and peaceful. This is explained in part by increasing relaxation as treatment progresses. It is clear to me in my work with people, though, that there is an added factor: while the more analytical and externally orientated side of the body is being stimulated there is a desire to talk, and there is a desire to retire into a deep place of innermost feelings, or of peacefulness, while the left side of the body is worked.

KNOWLEDGE AND WISDOM

When you have grasped the basics of how to use reflexology and where the reflexes are you will be able to stop thinking so hard about remembering what you have learned and start to tune in to the individual person you are working with. You will be able to learn from what their individual feet are showing you. Obviously it takes a while to familiarize yourself with the movements and the map of the feet. Even when you are quite confident about "where things are" you will still be learning if you are interested in and open to increasing your knowledge through experience. I learn all the time, both from my patient's experience of their individual problems and from other reflexologists.

When you feel comfortable giving a treatment without having to peer at the book or Illustrations 11 and 12 all the time you will be able to concentrate more on getting a feel for what you are doing. This is when you need to become aware of two aspects of the work: *what you do* and *how you do it.*

KNOWLEDGE

What you do is dependent on your taking the time to acquire the knowledge that will enable you to give a reflexology treatment. The information contained in this and other books will help you to learn the techniques of reflexology and the location and nature of the reflexes.

This body of knowledge includes information on reflexes to work for specific named conditions. Every reflexologist knows that we do not aim to treat any specific named condition, but rather treat the whole body and enable it to heal itself, thereby healing the specific problem. Even more importantly, a reflexologist should never *claim* to be able to cure any named condition, but rather to offer holistic help or treatment. Yet nearly every reflexology book contains information on which reflexes to work for certain common conditions. How you use (or misuse) this information is crucial. This is where wisdom comes in.

WISDOM

How you use this information is not learned from a textbook. It grows from the wisdom and experience you gain during the course of your life, from interaction with and empathy for others, from inspiration you may get from other people and other sources, and from your own personal development. Using this wisdom enables you to learn anew from every pair of feet you touch; to be aware that the charts on a two-dimensional piece of paper have to be applied to the unique pair of feet in your hands, which may differ considerably in structure from the ones illustrated on the chart. You have to be aware of the two-dimensional map of the reflexes but learn to apply it to the individual terrain you find whenever you give a treatment.

Using Knowledge and Wisdom

Equally important, *knowledge* allows you to work certain areas in addition to the whole to help the body alleviate certain problems; *wisdom* further adds an awareness that each person's experience of their illness is unique. For example, two people with asthma can have widely differing experiences. In this instance, wisdom directs you to check the information relating to areas to work for asthma, and then to find out how it applies to the individual pair of feet under your hands—to "see what stories the feet are telling you," as Eunice Ingham said so wisely.

Often people with a condition (our example here is asthma) will have tender and painful reflexes on some but not all of the expected areas. Further, they will have painful reflexes on points that are not in a charted relationship to asthma, but which are underlying the cause of the asthma in that person. Often the feet tell you things that people will not be aware of, or recognize themselves. *Never* discount the evidence of the feet because it does not fit the logic of your textbook knowledge.

So we see that knowledge of Illustrations 11 and 12 and theory of reflexology are important, but that awareness and an intuitive response to the individual person (wisdom) are equally essential.

Follow the Feet

Although reflexology has developed considerably in recent decades, the warmth and deep, yet straightforward, understanding provided by Eunice Ingham can teach you the essential approach. She shows you the "heart" of this work better than any other source. With a sound knowledge of physiology and a lifetime's dedication to finding out about and developing reflexology, Eunice Ingham was simply "in touch" with the people she worked with. She knew best how to help them to heal themselves. Throughout her books is the recurring phrase, and variations on it, "see what stories these feet can tell." If you have the wisdom to follow the lead of the feet in front of you as you work, and to respond accordingly with awareness, applying judiciously the knowledge you have learned, you will be doing good work. Details of Eunice Ingham's books are given on page 111.

IF YOUR PARTNER FINDS IT PAINFUL

Reflexology should be a relaxing and enjoyable experience: people will feel deeply relaxed or alternatively energized and stimulated according to their individual responses and needs. However, there can often be certain reflexes that trigger passing discomfort, tenderness or even sudden pain. When you meet these always stop and hold the area to relieve the pain and then give a massage to soothe your partner again. When you are able to continue working return to the area of discomfort, but work much more lightly, using less pressure so that it is not threatening to your partner. Never leave out an area of trouble because it is precisely those reflexes that most need treatment in order to release the tensions and toxins held in them.

If you cannot continue to do the reflexology techniques without causing pain then massage the reflex with a fingertip instead. If (rarely) you cannot do even that in a way your partner can bear then just hold the area in your hands for as long as seems right. Never leave anything out because it is too uncomfortable — find a way of *making* it comfortable.

WHY DO SOME REFLEX POINTS FEEL TENDER OR CONGESTED?

We say that these reflexes are out of balance. By this we mean that there is not a state of equilibrium where everything is able to function at optimum levels in that area of the body. This may be a passing state from day to day or evidence of a long-term problem.

We all experience states of tension in our bodies every day when we are hurried, under pressure, or feeling strained. These tensions will naturally release themselves during the course of the day if not added to. Each day we deal with and self-heal minor imbalances within our bodies. These minor stresses and strains clearly show up on the feet every time: the reflexes often show areas of tension so recent and minor that we were not even aware of them. If you are giving a reflexology treatment you help to release them as you work.

When an area of the foot remains tender or congested over several sessions this is likely to be imbalance of a longer duration. It is important that you know, and *crucial* that you convey to your partner, that the reflexes are very sensitive. "Trouble" found on the feet does not mean that the organ or body part that gives the reflex its name is diseased, though it may be stressed and benefit from relaxing the tension. It takes literally years of imbalance evidenced on the reflexes to build up disease at a reflex site.

Remember that if your partner is receiving medical care for any disorder you should only lightly massage the feet. A person should only receive reflexology after informing her doctor of her intentions.

COMMUNICATING — AND BEING AWARE OF WHAT YOU DO NOT KNOW

If your partner asks you which reflex it is that is so tender you must be aware, and communicate to them as well, that the reflexes overlap on the feet, just as the organs overlap in the body. The two-dimensional chart you are referring to is simplified and cannot accurately represent the complexity of the three-dimensional arrangement of the organs in your body. Because you cannot be certain, it would be incorrect to specifically say that it was the stomach or kidney reflex that was out of balance. It is fine to work that particular reflex in order to stimulate it because stimulating the circulation to that area releases any tension. It is wrong to give your partner information that may be inaccurate, which you cannot be sure about (remember Illustrations 11 and 12 are just guidelines and every pair of feet varies), and which could cause concern.

WORK FROM THE OUTSIDE IN

When working an area of imbalance, aim to release the tension and congestion from the outside in. If there is a tender place on the instep of the sole of the foot somewhere between the diaphragm and the waistline relating to the digestive system in the upper abdomen do not place your thumb in the center of the tender spot and rotate firmly on that spot. The correct way to proceed is to work around the edge of the perceived imbalance to try and release the congestion so that pressure and strain are taken away from that area. Gradually you will be able to work in toward the center, but always go from the outside in and not from the inside out.

Imagine a traffic jam. Pushing by the cars in the center of the jam to get out will only result in worse confusion and damage. The way to relieve such a jam is to move the cars at the outside edge so that the rest of the vehicles can filter out until the situation is resolved.

Also, do remember the value of *listening*. If your partner chooses to talk you will do as much good by really listening to her (without adding any of your opinions) as you will by massaging her feet.

14

THE ROUTINE

We have already looked at all areas of a reflexology treatment and the way in which we put these together. Here I am going to run through this again without the accompanying explanations so that you may refer to this section as a guide to giving a treatment.

Remember to check on the general health of your partner before you start. Remember, too, if someone has a problem on a limb (including the hands and feet) that the reflexes for these areas are called cross reflexes and they lie on the corresponding limb on the same side — see Illustration 2. You can also work out where the reflex for that part of the limb should lie along the outside of the foot (or hand) — see shoulder and knee reflex on Illustrations 11 and 12. But always massage the cross reflex because this can be very effective.

THE ORDER OF WORK

- Prepare yourself and what you need
- Position your partner
- Massage both feet a little, then cover the left one warmly

WORK THE RIGHT FOOT

- Massage the right foot thoroughly
- Thumb walk the toes and use other techniques as appropriate (1a–1e)
- Thumb walk the chest area on the ball of the foot and then finger walk on top (2a–2f)
- Work along the diaphragm (2d)
- Massage
- Thumb walk the abdominal area in the instep and use rotating and pin-pointing on the appropriate reflexes (3a–3c)
- Thumb walk the heel on the sole and work the sides of the heel for the pelvic area, using the appropriate techniques (4a–4c)
- Thumb walk or rotate along the reflex to the spine (5)
- Massage and warmly cover this foot

WORK THE LEFT FOOT

- Repeat the above exactly

TO COMPLETE

Massage both feet well at the end to finish with a sense of well-being and of completeness (use movements that embrace the whole foot).

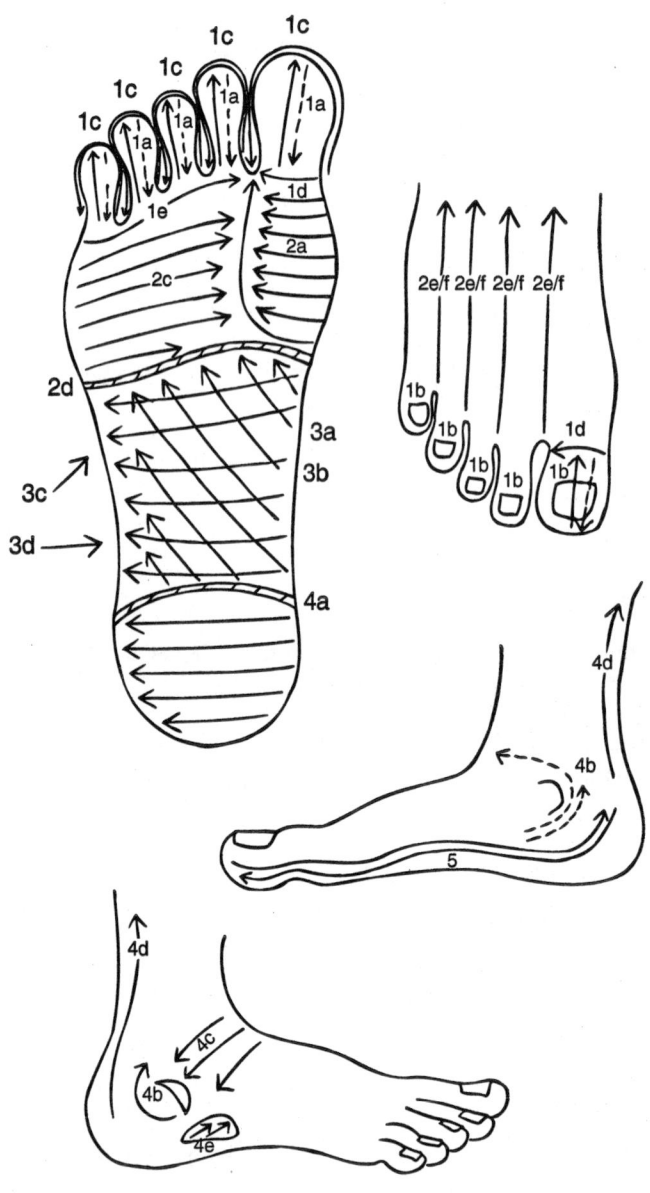

*Illustration 10
The Routine*

Note: Use massage techniques in the way that seems appropriate to you at the time and put in extra massage during the treatment of the reflexes. After something has hurt, always massage the area before continuing.

THE ROUTINE IN DETAIL — THE WAY AND DIRECTION IN WHICH TO WORK THE FEET

This is an explanation of Illustration 10.

- Prepare what you need (see Chapter 10) and yourself (see Chapter 11)
- Position your partner (see Chapter 10)
- Massage both feet a little, then cover the left one so that it is warm

WORK THE RIGHT FOOT

- Massage the right foot thoroughly
- Thumb walk the toes and use other techniques as appropriate
- When you want to give extra attention to a reflex, use rotation (see Chapter 12, page 70).

THE HEAD AND NECK AREA

THE BIG TOE

Hold the foot in your left hand on the outside of the foot, having your hand on the ball of the foot under the little toes: fingers on the top surface of the foot, thumb on the ball on the sole (the standard hold). Position your right hand on the inside of the foot under the big toe, with your fingers behind on the top of the foot, anchoring your hand to steady it and give you control.

Thumb walk up the back of the big toe from the base of the toe (its neck) to the top. Then continue over the top and down the front using your index finger to finger walk the front. Repeat this procedure twice, once on either side of your first path. This is necessary to cover the toe thoroughly because it is too wide to cover in one line.

Now thumb walk up the outside (medial side) of the big toe to the top. Then thumb walk up the inside (lateral side) of this toe, starting at the base and approaching it from the back. Thumb walk around the neck of the toe in two semi-circles: the back with the thumb and the front with the index finger. Then, using the pin-pointing technique (described in Chapter 12) find the pituitary reflex in the center of the lines of the toe print (this is often quite off-center in the toe).

Finally, change hands so that you hold the foot with the right hand on the ball under the big toe. With your left hand, approach from the front and thumb walk up the side of the big toe from the front (the lateral side next to the second toe). It is much easier to do than to read!

LITTLE TOES

Hold the foot with your left hand on the ball of the foot as you did for the big toe. Position your right hand also as before. Thumb walk up the back of the second toe to the top and finger walk (index finger) over the top and down the front of the toe. Now take your hand around to the front of the foot and tuck your thumb in between the second toe and the big toe and rotate on the web there. Then thumb walk up the side of the second toe to the top.

Finally, change hands again (as you did to finish on the big toe). Holding with your right hand, take your left hand around to the front of the foot and tuck it in between the second and third toes. Rotate on the web there and then thumb walk up this side of the second toe to the top.

Repeat this procedure exactly for each of the little toes in turn.

Now, with your right hand holding the foot on the ball under the big toe, thumb walk with your left hand along the ridge at the base of the little toes on the sole.

MASSAGE

Before you go on to the next area finish the area you are working on with massage.

THE CHEST AREA

BALL OF THE FOOT

Thumb walk the chest area. Hold the foot with your left hand as you did for the toes. With your right hand, thumb walk from the side of the foot across the ball, at the base of the big toe just under it, not under the other toes. Then repeat this just below the first line. Repeat again and continue to repeat until you meet the diaphragm, where the ball ends. This is rather like mowing the grass because your lines should touch each other without gaps, like the stripes on a lawn (see Illustration 10).

Next, with your right hand, hold the foot under the big toe (on the ball). With your left hand, thumb walk along underneath all the little toes on the ball of the foot. Then repeat this just below the first line and continue your lines like this until you reach the diaphragm line. (You are replicating under the little toes, from left to right, what you did under the big toe, right to left—lawn mowing. This is on the right foot; it will be the same, but with the direction reversed, on the other foot.) Thumb walk up each zone from the diaphragm to the toes.

THE CHEST ON THE TOP OF THE FOOT

With your left hand, hold the foot on the outside. With your right hand, thumb walk along the valley between the bones of the big and second toes, pressing your thumb more toward the right-hand side of the valley (the big toe side in this case). Do the same on the valley between the second and third toes; the third and fourth toes; and the fourth and fifth toes. Now work the same valleys again, this time with your middle finger (finger walking), and pressing more against the left-hand side of the valley (the other side from the one already covered). (2e)

Finally, using your three long fingers (second, third, and fourth), finger walk them all together from the base of the toes right down the foot to the ankle, working (strips) from one side to the other, covering the top of the foot thoroughly. (2f)

Work Along the Diaphragm

Thumb walk along the diaphragm line from either direction, or both. (2d)

Massage

Before going on to the next area finish the area you are working on with massage.

The Abdominal Area

Thumb walk the abdominal area in the instep and use rotating and pin-pointing on the appropriate reflexes. This area is also covered in strips, like a lawn.

With your left hand, hold the foot in the standard hold. With your right hand, thumb walk from the instep edge over the sole to the other side, just underneath the diaphragm. Repeat just below and continue your horizontal lines until you have covered the whole of the instep and come to the beginning of the heel.

Now thumb walk the same area again, this time with diagonal lines working from the instep edge diagonally upward to the diaphragm. Do the next line, each one becoming slightly longer, until halfway across the whole diagonal area where they begin to get shorter again.

You may have time to repeat these two ways of working (the horizontals and the diagonals), this time from the outside edge toward the instep. It is especially good to do this across the liver area. However, remember you cannot always do everything, and you have to make choices about what seems most appropriate on each occasion.

Specific Reflexes

Next there are some reflexes to work individually that are not reached any other way.

The Waistline

To identify the waistline, run your fingers down the outside of the foot until you feel and see the protruding end of the fifth metatarsal bone about halfway down. Take this prominence as your marker for the waistline; making an imaginary line right across the foot to the instep, this line is the waist.

The Adrenal Reflex

This is found by placing your right thumb horizontally just above the waistline on the instep and feeling forward, rotating, and under the tendon that runs down from the big toe. To identify this tendon, if it is not obvious, push the toes away from you toward the top surface of the foot with your holding hand (in this case the left one). With your right hand, run your fingertips gently across where the tendon lies in a line under the big toe until you can feel it. The kidney reflex is situated on the other (lateral) side of the tendon on a (horizontal) line with the adrenal, but covers a larger area, stretching down a little below the waistline. You do not need to rotate on this unless it seems to need extra attention.

The Gall Bladder Reflex

This reflex lies in zone four, halfway between the diaphragm and the waistline, or a little lower. Rotate on this reflex. To accurately find zone four this far down the foot, where it is narrower, take a line between the third and fourth toes and run down it until you come midway between the diaphragm and the waist.

The Ileo-Caecal Valve Reflex

This should be pin-pointed, as it is deep and can be hard to reach — be careful because it can also be very tender. To find it, feel below that end of the metatarsal bone that marks the waistline and feel the hollow that lies below it. Horizontally on a line with this, but in zone four (under the gall bladder), is the reflex to be pin-pointed.

The Colon Reflex

Thumb walk up the colon with your left hand (right hand holding) as it runs from the heel line up and alongside (just outside but overlapping) the ileo-caecal valve and then across the transverse colon on and just above the waist.

The Bladder Reflex

This reflex does not need specific working unless it shows imbalance. It is found where the spine and heel line intersect.

Massage

Before going on finish the area you are working on with massage.

The Pelvic Area

Thumb walk the heel on the sole and work the sides of the heel for the pelvic area using the appropriate techniques. On the sole, hold with your left hand and thumb walk with your right, walk horizontal lines, as before, from the heel line down until you reach the end of the heel. Or you may carefully run the knuckle of your index finger down each zone from the heel line to the end.

On the outside of the foot is the reflex to the gonads (ovaries or testes), located midway along a line running between the center of the top of the ankle bone and the right angle of the heel. Rotate this. Then thumb or finger walk across the top of the ankle where the foot joins the leg (you can see a crease at this point if you push the foot up and back toward the leg). Do this in three strips to cover the lower lymph reflex thoroughly. Then work with your fingertips rotating, feeling in all around the ankle bone. The top of the ankle is also the reflex to the fallopian tubes or vas deferens.

Find the reflex to the uterus or prostate on the inside of the heel in exactly the same way as you did the gonads on the outside. Work it by rotating. Then work around the inner ankle bone as you did the outer.

Using your middle finger, walk up behind the ankle bones and up the sides of both legs a little way. Finally, work the soft triangle to be found on the outside of the heel behind or below the protruding metatarsal bone.

THE SPINE

Thumb walk or rotate along the reflex to the spine. Work from the top of the big toe (the crown of the head) down the side of the toe (the cervical spine begins beside the root of the nail, by the first toe joint) down the neck of the toe (and the neck reflex) on the same line. Continue down the foot, following the edge up the arch of the instep and down it again to the heel line. Here the spinal line runs along just above the upper edge of the bony part of the heel, where there is some "give." It finishes by curving around below the ankle (following the most yielding part on the edge of the bone) ending in the reflex to the coccyx — see Illustrations 11 and 12.

Note: Remember to use rotation whenever you want to give extra attention to a reflex.

MASSAGE

Finish with massage, and then cover this foot warmly.

THE LEFT FOOT

On the left foot repeat all of the above exactly, only reverse left and right to match the shape of the left foot (instep on your left here rather than on your right), as in a mirror image. Don't think about it —follow the shape of the feet and you will do it naturally. Do not let the words mix you up.

TO COMPLETE

Massage both feet well at the end to finish with a sense of well-being and completeness (use movements that embrace the whole foot).

It is a good idea to draw your own Illustrations 11 and 12 from those in this book. This will help you learn where the reflexes are. You will also then have your own illustrations to place alongside these directions as you work.

A professional reflexology session takes about an hour. When you are learning it can seem to take ages. Do not worry if it takes more than an hour, but aim to contain it within an hour and a half or your partner may have too much. Allow about half an hour for each foot while you are learning. A professional has to fit everything into the hour — from entering the room to leaving it — so it works out as less time per foot.

Remember you cannot always do everything and will have to choose what to spend the time on. *However, always cover the whole of the feet in some way.*

CASE STUDIES

CASE ONE: SHORT-TERM INJURY

Ken is a middle-aged company chairman. He has a demanding desk job, and attends a gym once a week to try to compensate for a sedentary and stressful lifestyle. He pulled a muscle in his left shoulder one week; three days later he came to me with his neck and shoulders seized up. He was unable to turn his head.

This man did not have an interest in complementary medicine and came rather reluctantly by recommendation. During the first part of the treatment I worked while we had an interesting conversation about unrelated subjects. After twenty minutes he suddenly sat up and asked "Is it meant to work right away?" By the end of the session Ken was able to move fairly freely and felt quite comfortable. The following day I received a very good bottle of wine and the message that he was completely restored to normal!

Case Two: Irritable Bowel Syndrome (IBS)

Ralph is thirty-eight years old. Having had chronic IBS for eighteen months he came to me when the bowel had ruptured and was bleeding. After one treatment there was no more bleeding. The condition continued to heal and improve over the next few months while he received weekly treatments.

Case Three: Repetitive Strain Injury

Jessica is a thirty-six-year-old woman. Working at a computer for long periods most days Jessica had developed floaters in her eyes that seemed like cobwebs across her vision. She commented on how well she felt at the end of the first treatment. After two weeks Jessica reported that it was working and the floaters in her eyes were definitely less! By the end of two months the condition had cleared completely.

Case Four: Asthma

Timmy is a nine-year-old boy. His life was seriously restricted by recurrent and distressing asthma attacks. The reflexes of the respiratory system were very congested; all the main endocrine glands were out of balance and very painful, as was the ileo-caecal valve. I gave him weekly treatments of suitable duration for a child (shorter than for an adult). In four sessions the reflexes were much less tender, with improvement in Timmy's breathing. His asthma attacks were less severe. In four months the asthma had completely cleared.

Case Five: Sinusitis

Nina is a woman in her early twenties. She has had problems with her sinuses since childhood. The reflexes on all the toes were very congested and painful. After the first session Nina developed a heavy cold, but this had cleared by the second week of treatment and the sinuses were much clearer. By the fourth treatment Nina's sinuses were quite clear and she continued to receive treatment for an additional few weeks.

CASE SIX: ANGELA

The following case is an in-depth working case study. Angela is a fifty-eight-year-old woman.

PRESENTING PROBLEMS

The patient had a viral infection in the spring that dragged on for six weeks, started to clear up, and then came back again. Three months later, when she came to me she was still feeling very low.

MEDICAL HISTORY

Angela has had high blood pressure for about six years, and has been on hormone replacement therapy (HRT) for six months following menopause. Concerned about her weight being too high, the doctor advised her to cut down on food. She does not want to do this because she has a naturally small appetite. Angela has had her metabolism checked, which her doctor says showed normal thyroid activity and no problems.

Her circulation could be better: she has cold hands and feet. Her digestive system is generally fine, but Angela often wakes in the morning with an uncomfortable feeling of fullness, as if she had just eaten a large meal.

Angela has had some difficulty with her breathing, but does not feel troubled by it because she lives within her limits. Her doctor diagnosed asthma and prescribed an inhaler, which she does not use because she puts her breathlessness down to the polluted environment of her hometown (which is in a steep river basin so the air is contained, and it has heavy traffic going through it).

Angela wears glasses because her eyes are different from each other. She sometimes has headaches and occasional migraines when she is very tired or if she is affected by flashing lights (for instance driving in bright sunlight down a tree-lined road).

Following the birth of one of her children Angela's chronic pelvic/back trouble was finally relieved by visits to a chiropractor. She broke her left ankle one and a half years ago.

Family History and Lifestyle

Angela lives with her husband, a landscape gardener. He is now working again after a prolonged period of serious illness eight years ago when he had two heart attacks and had to give up work. This was a very difficult time for Angela, both in caring for her husband and because of financial worries. Angela has three children, all grown, and five grandchildren, two of whom she sees regularly and looks after once a week. Both her parents are still living but are very old and rather senile.

Angela has had a busy and interesting life, at one time working as an office manager for a medical practice and then owning and running her own upscale delicatessen (which she had to sell when her husband was ill). Her current occupations are her family, home, and garden. Angela attends art and pottery classes and paints at home.

She enjoys good food and cooking, especially Italian and Thai cuisine, and has a small but healthy diet. She says she has a very sweet tooth, which is not pandered to. Angela drinks mineral water, tea, coffee, and sometimes herb tea, but says that she does not drink enough water because she does not like the taste of tap water. She enjoys drinking wine, in moderation, and sometimes whiskey.

Angela falls asleep easily but does not sleep very well. She is a light sleeper and wakes easily, often staying awake worrying. She dreams quite a lot and has a recurring nightmare of losing one of the children.

Emotional History

Angela has been under enormous strain for some years following her husband's long-term illness. She feels that she still carries the effects of that, although now their life is quite satisfactory and comfortable. She sometimes suffers from stress. She usually knows the cause, and feels she generally deals with stress well. She can also get angry.

Observation

Angela seems relaxed, with a friendly and interested manner. She is of medium height and well rounded, but not especially large. She has a little redness in the cheeks, her hair is fine, and her skin is inclined to be dry.

Observation of the feet Angela's feet are broad, having kept their shape, though the toes are quite curled under. There is dry skin all over the soles and on the plantar heels particularly, where the skin is purple and mottled with lots of tiny cracks. She has a lot of hard skin, especially a ridge on the right thyroid helper reflex and on the left big toe lateral to the pituitary reflex. There is a seed corn on the right foot on the reflex to the small intestine, and two on the left foot under the second toe, on the stomach meridian, and on the chest reflex. In both cases these are lying in the second zone.

Treatment Plan

We decided on full treatment, aiming to boost the body's functioning after a debilitating illness, and also to promote relaxation and bring down the blood pressure levels. The glands were to be worked to check the state of their reflexes and to stimulate them if necessary to help restore health after the illness. I also had in mind a boost to the body's hormone functioning because Angela is on HRT, and particularly the thyroid to assist her metabolism rate if necessary, and the pancreas because of her "sweet tooth." The left eye showed more imbalance because there was a sharp shooting pain through the eye reflex on first contact. This reflex remained tender for a long time.

I need to check the digestive and urinary systems, as Angela acknowledges that she does not drink enough fluid. The second zone needs to be thoroughly checked and worked because a number of these findings lie on it or are related to the stomach meridian (eyes, digestive system, and sweet tooth).

Recommendation

I recommended an initial course of eight sessions, to be reviewed as we went along to see what responses had occurred.

Treatment 1: Initial Findings

There was a great deal of tension and pain in the toes, especially on the reflexes to the eyes and the side of neck/mastoid bone (process) on the left big toe. Angela experienced a very sharp, shooting pain on this reflex. The pituitary reflex was painful and there was a lot of pain on the eye/ear helper ridge under the toes. The thyroid helper reflex was painful and very congested to the touch. The whole chest area was congested.

The diaphragm and the reflex to the adrenal gland on the left foot were tender. There was evidence of poor tone right across the abdominal area. The descending and sigmoid colon was a little tender and the sigmoid flexure was very tender. Also taken into account and worked were the plantar heels (dry, cracked, and purple) and the seed corns on the stomach meridian on the second zone on both feet.

Everything was more painful on the left foot than on the right.

TREATMENT 2

Feedback Angela arrived very pleased, saying that her blood pressure had been tested and had been normal in the first time for years, and after only one treatment! She also said that she had more energy and was not as tired.

Findings The toes were slightly less painful than on the first session. The other reflexes responded similarly to last time, with the thyroid helper, diaphragm, and sigmoid colon being the most significantly tender, and the chest area was very congested.

TREATMENT 3

Feedback Angela arrived saying that she felt tired and depleted after having her elderly parents — who need a great deal of attention — for the weekend and a large family party with lots of cooking to do.

Findings The neck reflexes were much more painful than last time, showing that she had been very tense. As soon as I started to work on the toes her tummy began to rumble because the tension was released; this often happens but was particularly pronounced today. Otherwise the feet were much the same as previously.

TREATMENTS 4 – 6

Feedback Angela noticed a consistent improvement in her energy levels and each week said that she was feeling better. Her blood pressure was still good.

Findings There was no noticeable improvement in the state of the reflexes, although she was feeling much better. This does not worry me because we are dealing with long-standing problems that will probably take a while to shift.

The important thing is that the patient is experiencing an improvement in her health.

TREATMENTS 7 – 11

By the time Angela stopped coming weekly during the summer she was feeling that she was in very good health (her words) and experiencing plenty of energy. The reflexes had improved gradually, the chest area being the main reflex to show continued low level imbalance. The reflexes to the neck were often painful because that is one of the primary areas where she takes on stress. The pain came and went from week to week and was not consistent. The heaviness in the digestive system in the mornings improved to a point where she seldom experienced it.

TREATMENTS 12 – 18

Angela came back four months later, following her vacation and then a worrying and tiring period of coping with family problems. She felt very depleted and her reflexes held a lot of pain. They were on a whole seriously out of balance.

Usually when a patient returns for a second course of treatment after a gap the body responds more readily. Progress is faster because the body/mind/spirit recognizes the improved state of well-being that it experienced before. In this case progress was actually quite slow and it took four or five weeks for Angela to begin to pick up again. This tells me that she had been under a lot of strain in the previous two months that had taken its toll.

Feedback During the last month of weekly treatments Angela made steady progress and felt restored to equilibrium. She decided that she would like to come monthly for treatment to help maintain her good state of health.

SUMMARY

I anticipate that it should be possible to establish and maintain a greatly improved state of well-being on a permanent basis. This patient wishes to continue with treatment for the time being as she has benefited greatly from it.

Angela's case clearly illustrates how a person with a healthy lifestyle who is fundamentally happy and satisfied within herself can experience a breakdown of health under extreme stress. I was surprised that her blood pressure responded immediately to the release of locked-in tension in her body through an initial reflexology treatment.

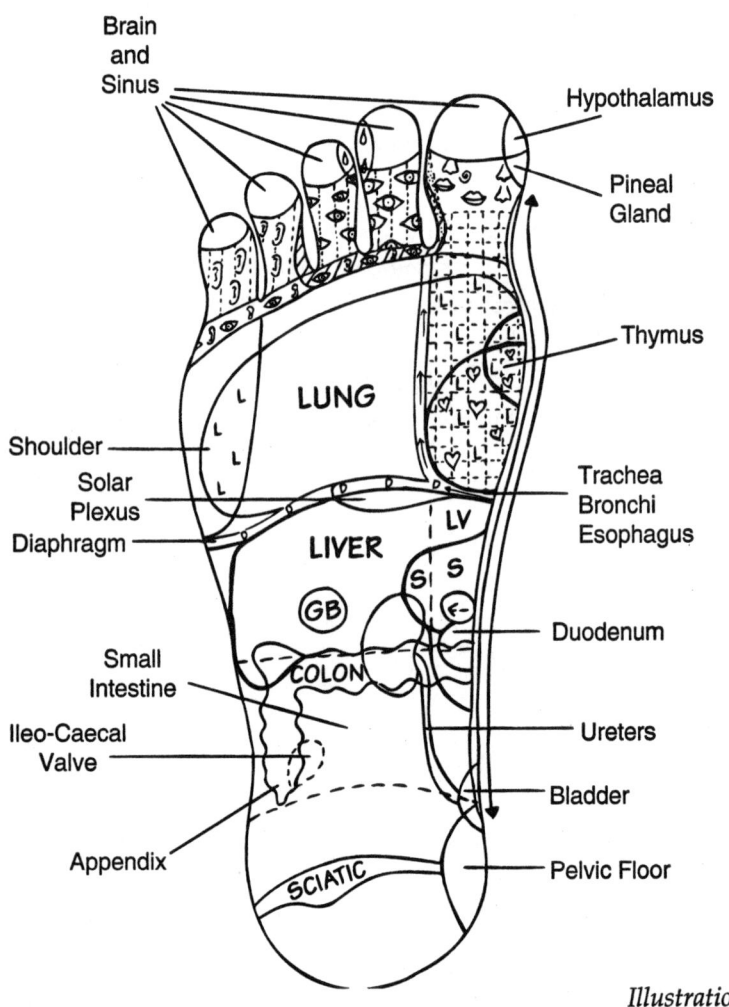

Illustration 11

Key for Figures 11 and 12:

👁 eyes	💧 lachrymal gland	[P] parathyroid
⤴ ears	∴ side of neck	/// eustacian tube
👃 nose	⋮⋮⋮ neck	☉ pituitary gland
👄 mouth	[ ] thyroid	T thymus

DISCOVER REFLEXOLOGY 109

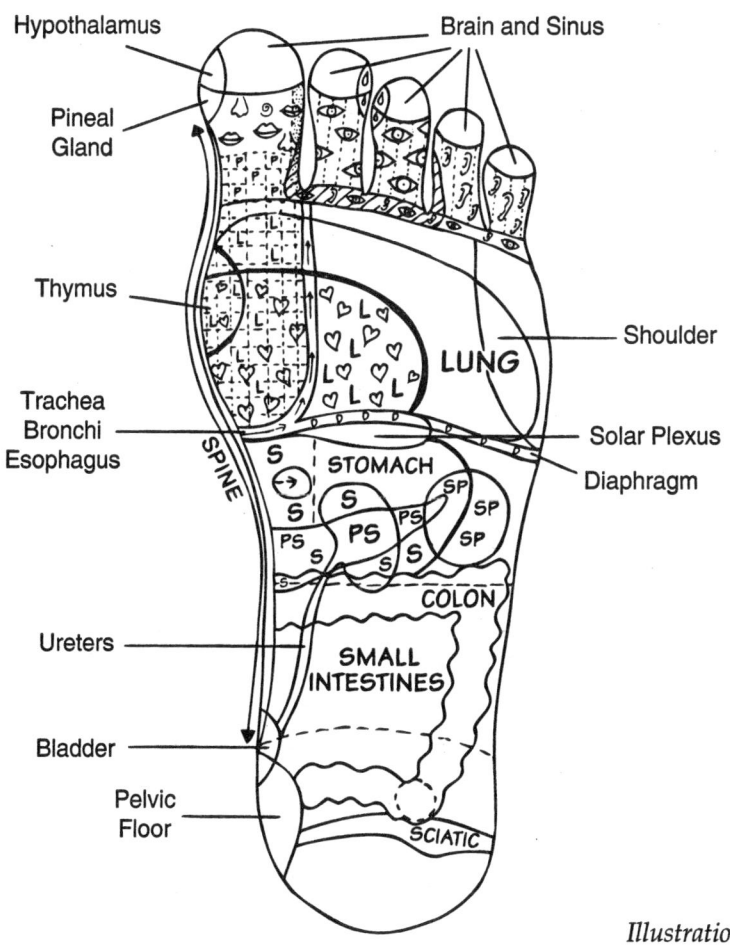

Illustration 12

Key (continued):

↑ trachea, bronchi, esopagus	**SP** spleen	**GB** gall bladder
L lungs	**PS** pancreas	**LV** liver
♡ heart	🫘 kidneys	**D** diaphragm
S stomach	⊖ adrenal glands	

110 DISCOVER REFLEXOLOGY

Illustration 13

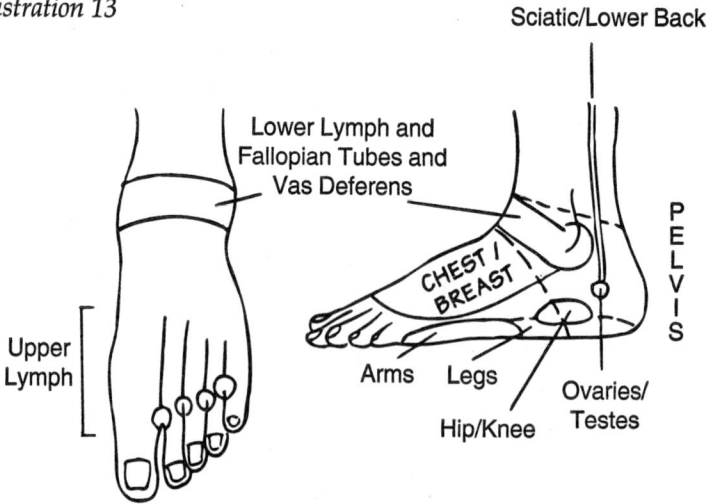

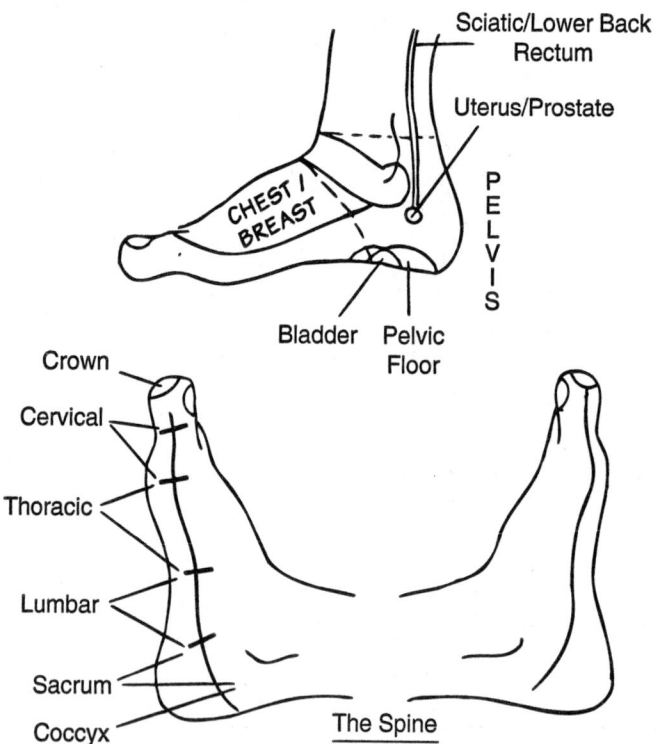

RECOMMENDED READING

The following titles are the best books offering a comprehensive understanding of reflexology.

Dougans, Inge and Ellis, Suzanne, *The Art of Reflexology*, London: Element Books, 1992.

Gillanders, Ann, *Reflexology: The Ancient Answer to Modern Ailments*, Bristol: J. W. Arrowsmith, 1987.

Ingham, Eunice, *Stories the Feet Can Tell Thru Reflexology and Stories the Feet Have Told Thru Reflexology*, USA: Ingham Publishing, 1984.

Lambert, Mary C., *Finding Your Feet*, London: M & J Lambert, 1988.

Stormer, Chris, *Reflexology: the Definitive Guide*, London: Headline Hodder & Stoughton, 1995.

Further Reading

Byers, Dwight, *Better Health with Foot Reflexology*, USA: Ingham Publishing, 1983.

Carter, Mildred, *Hand Reflexology*, New York: Parker Publishing, 1975.

Gillanders, Ann, *Reflexology — the Theory and Practice*, England: Jenny Lee Publishing Services, 1994.

Saint-Pierre, Gaston and Shapiro, Debbie, *The Metamorphic Technique*, London: Element Books, 1982.

Stormer, Chris, *The Language of the Feet*, London: Headline Hodder and Stoughton, 1995.

General Books

Chappell, Peter, *Emotional Healing with Homeopathy*, London: Element Books, 1994.

Hay, Louise, *You Can Heal Your Life*, London: Eden Grove Editions, 1984.

Holt, John, *How Children Fail*, London: Penguin, 1969.

Liedloff, Jean, *The Continuum Concept*, London: Arkana, 1989.

Mendelssohn, Dr. Robert S., *Confessions of a Medical Heretic*, USA: Warner Books, 1979.

Miller, Alice, *Banished Knowledge*, London: Virago, 1990.

Miller, Alice, *The Drama of Being a Child*, London: Virago, 1979.

Page, Dr. Christine R., *Frontiers of Health*, Saffron Walden: C. W. Daniel, 1992.

Satir, Virginia, *The New Peoplemaking*, USA: Science and Behavior Books, 1988.

INDEX

Abdominal reflex area, 79, 94–95
Acupuncture, 1–2, 17–18
Adrenal reflex, 95
Almond oil, 56
Alternative medicine, 28
Ankle loosening, and foot massage, 61, 63
Ankle rotation, and foot massage, 61, 62
Ankle stretch, and foot massage, 62
Arms, 12, 14, 88
Arrowroot, 55

Babies, and reflexology, 15
Baby powder, 55
Balanced state, 46
Barefoot doctors of China, 17–18
Bladder reflex, 96
Blanket, for warmth, 55
Blockage in energy flow, 26
Blood circulation, 14, 22, 39
Body, represented on feet, 9–10, 12–14
Body temperature, during reflexology, 55

Bowel movements, increased, as healing reaction, 41
Brain, right and left sides, 80
Byers, Dwight, 18

Calendula lotion, 55–56
Callouses, 52
Case studies, 99–107
Caterpillar walking technique, and reflexology, 68–69, 70
Cellular memory, 42–43
Change, 4, 19, 25–27, 30, 33
Chemical additives in food, 5, 6
Chest reflex area, 79, 93–94
Ch'i (life force), 17
Children, and reflexology, 15, 21
China, ancient, and foot treatments, 1–2, 16, 17
Circulation. *See* Blood circulation
Coccyx reflex, 98
Colon reflex, 96
Common cold, 35
  as healing reaction, 41
Communication, importance of, 46, 50, 52, 86–87
Compassion, 33

Conditions, named, 29–30, 54, 83
Corns, 52
Cross reflexes, 14, 88
Cure, concept of, 43–44

Deposits of waste material, 14
Diabetics, and reflexology treatments, 47, 53–54
Diagnosis, and reflexology, 28
Diaphragm, and foot massage, 61, 64–65
Discomfort, 85. *See also* Tenderness
Dis-ease and disease, 24–25, 29–30, 34
and trauma, 31–37
Distress, 7–8
Dougans, Inge, 19
Dreams, as healing reaction, 41

Effects of treatment, 14–15, 21–23, 38–44
Effleurage and foot massage, 58, 59
Egypt, ancient, and foot treatments, 16
Elderly, and treatments, 21
Electromagnetic energy, 10
Emotions
and reflexology, 42–43
physical manifestations, 2, 3, 7–8, 26, 32–33, 42–43
Energy and energy flow, 10–11, 14, 22, 43–44, 46, 73
along spine, 73
blockage, 26
Equipment and supplies, for reflexology, 55–56
Essential oils, 56
Europe, and pressure point therapy, 18

Fallopian tubes reflex, 97
Feet
embarrassment about, 56
texture and color, 78
Finger walking technique, and reflexology, 70
Fitzgerald, Dr. William, 18, 76
Five Element acupuncture, 17–18
Food and health, 4–6
Foot massage, 11, 57–66, 80
techniques, 58–66
Frequency of treatment, 23, 47–48
Fruit, 5–6

Gall bladder reflex, 96
Gonads reflex, 97

Hand support
and foot massage, 58–59
and reflexology, 67–68
Harvey, William, 11
Head reflex area, 78–79, 91–93
Headache, 52, 74
as healing reaction, 41
Healing crisis, 40–42
Healing reactions, 40–42
Health, 24–30
and food, 4–6
and reflexology, 1–8
Holding technique, and reflexology, 72
Holistic aspects of reflexology, 2, 45–48
Homeostasis, 46
"Hook in and back up" technique, and reflexology, 72

Ileo-caecal valve reflex, 79, 96
Imbalance, visual signs of, 52

India, ancient, and foot treatments, 16
Infection protection, 52, 54, 57
Ingham, Eunice, 18, 84–85
Interruptions during reflexology, 56

Kidney reflex, 95
Kneading, and foot massage, 61, 62–63
Knee-jerk reflex, 11
Knowledge, 83, 84

Lawn mowing technique, and reflexology, 93
Left brain, 80
Legs, 12, 14, 88
Length of treatment, 21, 98
Life force, 17, 19
Limbs (arms and legs), 12, 14, 88
Listening, importance of, 87
Liver function, 3
Lowered defenses, 39–40
Lymph circulation, 14, 22
Lymph reflex, 97

Malnutrition, 6
Massage. *See* Foot massage
Materials, for reflexology, 55–56
Medical history, personal, 21, 47
Meridian theory, 76
Meridians, 76, 77
Metamorphic Technique (Metamorphosis), 19
Muscles, 14, 22

Natural laws, 4
Neck reflex area, 78–79, 91–93
North American Indians, and foot massage, 16
Number of treatments, 15, 47–48

Oils, 55, 56
Order of work. *See* Sequence of treatment
Ovaries reflex, 97

Pain, 85. *See also* Tenderness
Patient–practitioner cooperation, 22, 23, 45–46, 50, 86–87
Pelvic reflex area, 79, 96–97
Physics, 10
Pin-pointing technique, and reflexology, 70–71
Pituitary reflex, 92
Position during reflexology, 54–55
Powder, 55
Pressure therapy, 18
Prostate reflex, 97

Rash, as healing reaction, 41
Reflexes, 11, 17, 78–80, 91–98
  congested, 85–86
Reflexologist, professional, 50–51
  choosing, 48
Reflexology
  benefits, 21, 39–40
  case studies, 99–107
  effects, 14–15, 38–44
  and health, 1–8
  history, 1–2, 16–19
  holistic aspects, 2, 45–48
  physiological effects, 14, 38–39
  psychosomatic effects, 43
  techniques, 67–81, 88–98
  treatments, 14–15, 21–23, 38–44, 53–56, 67–81, 88–98
Responsibility for health, 36
Right brain, 80

Rotating technique, and reflexology, 70
Rotation of toes, and foot massage, 63
Routine, for reflexology treatment, 80–81, 88–98

Saint Augustine, 4
St. John, Robert, 19
Self-healing, 22, 25, 34–36
Self-help reflexology treatments, 48, 51–52, 53–56
Self-observation, 28, 31–32
Sequence of treatment, 80–81, 88–98
Shiatsu, 17
Side to side movements, and foot massage, 61, 63
Skin
  broken, and infection, 52, 54
  hard, 52
  rash, as healing reaction, 41
Solar plexus, and foot massage, 61, 65
Spinal twist, and foot massage, 61, 63–64
Spine, 19
  reflex area, 79, 97–98
Spreading movements, and foot massage, 60, 61, 62
Stimulating movements, and foot massage, 61, 63
Stress, 8
Stroking movements, and foot massage, 58, 59
Supporting hand
  and foot massage, 58–59
  and reflexology, 67–68

Talcum powder, 55
Talking during treatment, 47, 80

Techniques, 67–81, 88–98. *See also specific techniques*
Tenderness, 21, 70, 72, 85–86
  and reflex points, 15, 85–86
Tennis elbow, 14
Tension, 14, 15, 22–23
Testes reflex, 97
Thumb walking technique, and reflexology, 68–69, 70
Toe rotation, and foot massage, 63
Towel, to cover foot, 55
Toxins, 7, 40
Transverse zones, 76, 77, 78
Trauma, 23
  and disease, 31–37
Treatments, 14–15, 21–23, 38–44, 53–56, 67–81, 88–98
  effects, 15, 21–23, 38–44
  frequency, 23, 47–48
  length, 21, 98
  number needed, 15, 47–48
  sequence, 80–81, 88–98
Truth, 37

Up and down movements, and foot massage, 61, 63
Urination, increased, as healing reaction, 41
Uterus reflex, 97

Vegetable oils, 56
Verrucas, 52

Waistline reflex, 81, 95
Warmth during reflexology, 55
Waste products, 14
Will to live, 35
Wisdom, 83–84

Zone theory, 18, 76
Zones, 75, 76, 78

OTHER ULYSSES PRESS HEALTH TITLES

ANXIETY AND DEPRESSION: A NATURAL APPROACH
Shirley Trickett

> By addressing the patient's total health from a physical *and* mental standpoint, *Anxiety and Depression: A Natural Approach* avoids the failure of traditional medical treatment. With specific suggestions on diet, breathing, relaxation, bio-feedback, and exercise, the program helps sufferers empower themselves to prevent further discomfort. $8.95

THE BOOK OF KOMBUCHA
Beth Ann Petro

> *The Book of Kombucha* explains the health benefits of the "tea mushroom" while answering the concerns surrounding this alternative health treatment. Draws on up-to-date research and explains how to grow and use Kombucha. $11.95

BREAKING THE AGE BARRIER:
STAYING YOUNG, HEALTHY AND VIBRANT
Helen Franks

> Drawing on the latest medical research, *Breaking the Age Barrier* explains how the proper lifestyle can stop the aging process and make you feel youthful and vital. $12.95

COUNT OUT CHOLESTEROL
Art Ulene, M.D. and Val Ulene, M.D.

> Complete with counter and detailed dietary plan, this companion resource to the *Count Out Cholesterol Cookbook* shows how to design a cholesterol-lowering program that's right for you. $12.95

COUNT OUT CHOLESTEROL COOKBOOK
Art Ulene, M.D. and Val Ulene, M.D.

> A companion guide to *Count Out Cholesterol*, this book shows you how to bring your cholesterol levels down with the help of 250 gourmet recipes. $14.95

DISCOVER MEDITATION: A FIRST-STEP GUIDE TO BETTER HEALTH
Doriel Hall

> *Discover Meditation* leads the reader step by step through a journey of discovery into this ancient discipline. Chapters address everything from physical positioning and breathing techniques to focusing the mind and achieving self-knowledge. $8.95

DISCOVER OSTEOPATHY: A FIRST-STEP GUIDE TO BETTER HEALTH
Peta Sneddon and Paolo Coseschi

> In *Discover Osteopathy*, two practicing osteopaths explain simply and lucidly the basic principles of osteopathy, when to visit an osteopath, and how osteopathy works. Specific chapters detail osteopathic techniques, and special sections look at the application of these therapies in areas like pregnancy, childbirth, and even dentistry. $8.95

DISCOVER REFLEXOLOGY: A FIRST-STEP GUIDE TO BETTER HEALTH
Rosalind Oxenford

> *Discover Reflexology* relates this ancient tradition to its historical context within Chinese medicine and to the modern understanding of holistic health programs that address body, mind, and spirit. This book empowers the beginner to incorporate the therapy into his or her own personal program of good health. $8.95

DISCOVERY PLAY
Art Ulene, M.D. and Steven Shelov, M.D.

> This book guides parents through the first three years of their child's life, offering play activity with a special emphasis on nurturing self-esteem. $9.95

IRRITABLE BOWEL SYNDROME: A NATURAL APPROACH
Rosemary Nicol

> This book offers a natural approach to a problem millions of sufferers have. The author clearly defines the symptoms and offers a dietary and stress-reduction program for relieving the effects of this disease. $9.95

KNOW YOUR BODY: THE ATLAS OF ANATOMY
Introduction by Trevor Weston, M.D.

> Designed to provide a comprehensive and concise guide to the structure of the human body, *Know Your Body* offers more than 250 color illustrations. An easy-to-follow road map of the human body. $12.95

LAST WISHES: A HANDBOOK TO GUIDE YOUR SURVIVORS
Lucinda Page Knox, M.S.W. and Michael D. Knox, Ph.D.

> A simple do-it-yourself workbook, *Last Wishes* helps people put their affairs in order and eases the burden on their survivors. It allows them to plan their own funeral and leave final instructions for survivors. $12.95

LOSE WEIGHT WITH DR. ART ULENE
Art Ulene, M.D.

> This best-selling weight-loss book offers a 28-day program for taking off the pounds and keeping them off forever. $12.95

MOOD FOODS
William Vayda

> *Mood Foods* shows how the foods you eat can influence your emotions, behavior, and personality. It also explains how a proper diet can help to alleviate such common complaints as PMS, hyperactivity, mood swings, and stress. $9.95

PANIC ATTACKS: A NATURAL APPROACH
Shirley Trickett

> Addresses the problem of panic attacks using a holistic approach. Focusing on diet and relaxation, the book helps you prevent future attacks. $8.95

THE VITAMIN STRATEGY
Art Ulene, M.D. and Val Ulene, M.D.

> A game plan for good health, this book helps readers design a vitamin and mineral program tailored to their individual needs. $11.95

YOUR NATURAL PREGNANCY: A GUIDE TO COMPLEMENTARY THERAPIES
Anne Charlish

> This timely book brings together the many complementary therapies such as aromatherapy, massage, homeopathy, acupressure, herbal medicine, and meditation, that can benefit pregnant women. $16.95

To order these or other Ulysses Press books call 800-377-2542 or write to Ulysses Press, P.O. Box 3440, Berkeley, CA 94703-3440. All retail orders are shipped free of charge. California residents must include sales tax. Allow two to three weeks for delivery.

Rosalind Oxenford M.A.R. practices and teaches reflexology in Bath, where whe has her own School of Reflexology.